The International Library of Psychology

THE ART

INTERROGATION

Founded by C. K. Ogden

The International Library of Psychology

INDIVIDUAL DIFFERENCES
In 21 Volumes

THE ART OF INTERROGATION

Studies in the Principles of Mental Tests and Examinations

E R HAMILTON

Introduction by C Spearman

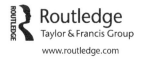

Routledge
Taylor & Francis Group
www.routledge.com

First published in 1929 by
Kegan Paul, Trench, Trubner & Co., Ltd.

Published in 2001 by
Routledge
2 Park Square, Milton Park, Abingdon, Oxfordshire OX14 4RN
711 Third Avenue, New York, NY 10017

First issued in paperback 2014

Routledge is an imprint of the Taylor and Francis Group, an informa business

The publishers have made every effort to contact authors/copyright holders
of the works reprinted in the *International Library of Psychology*.
This has not been possible in every case, however, and we would
welcome correspondence from those individuals/companies
we have been unable to trace.

British Library Cataloguing in Publication Data
A CIP catalogue record for this book
is available from the British Library

The Art of Interrogation
ISBN 0415-21058-5
Individual Differences: 21 Volumes
ISBN 0415-21130-1
The International Library of Psychology: 204 Volumes
ISBN 0415-19132-7

ISBN 978-1-138-88252-2 (pbk)
ISBN 978-0-415-21058-4 (hbk)

To

MY FATHER AND MOTHER

CONTENTS

INTRODUCTION

IF there is anything as old as the first human intercourse and yet as modern as the correspondence columns in the newspapers, anything that can give to the recipient exquisite delight or inflict unendurable pain, anything that will probably bring forth truth and yet is unequalled for generating falsehood—surely it is the asking of a question. Heavily fraught with interest, then, is the topic of " interrogation " that has been chosen for the following small volume, to which I have so kindly been invited to contribute a few opening words.

The aspects of the topic which the author has chosen to delineate on the present occasion are : first and foremost the so-called " mental tests " ; and then examinations—in both the old style and the new ; and finally the questioning that is performed by the teacher in the class-room. Assuredly, at least the first and second of these doings have earned and obtained the liveliest concern, not only of those who busy themselves with the momentous task of educating the young, but also of those who have the still more arduous duty of fitting each individual into his or her proper place in the constitution of society.

Now on these subjects, especially the tests and the examinations, the present author undoubtedly offers us here the fruit of a very long, careful, and penetrating study. To his undertaking he has brought an exceptional equipment of expert knowledge combined with an unusually broad outlook ; to which advantages must be added the gift of pleasing and lucid exposition. All those very numerous persons whom duty or curiosity may incline to orient themselves in these subjects—which without such aid present nowadays extraordinary difficulties—will find in this little book just the effective and enjoyable guidance of which they stand in need.

But such a popularising mission of the book is incidental rather than primary. Its first aim is, rather, to make a serious donation to exact science, to clear up much that has been nebulous even in the writings of the leading authorities, and to disentangle much that is now unprogressively controversial. And without suggesting that this volume will establish a millennium-day from which time onwards we shall all see all things eye to eye, one may venture to prophesy that it will at least assist in this desirable direction.

C. SPEARMAN.

PREFACE

THE methods of gauging mental qualities must always form one of the main themes of educational psychology. For, not only does the practice of education demand the continual exploration of the minds of pupils, but any theory of education, since it necessarily presupposes a theory of mental action, must be sanctioned by the results of adequate psychological testing. But whilst recent writings on educational psychology make abundant reference to mental testing, the basic principles of interpretation of tests are only rarely and scantily treated. If this book does something to further the establishment of such principles, one of its chief aims will have been achieved.

Though examinations are of such long standing, and intimately affect so many people, the critical survey of the principles governing their use has but seldom been seriously attempted. Yet it was inevitable that the great development of mental tests in recent years should kindle interest in the possibility of reforming examinations. The resulting attempts at reform have now proceeded far enough to be, in their turn, criticized, and with such criticism much of this book is, directly or indirectly, concerned.

The book has been kept as free as possible from technical terms, and is entirely free from the statistical machinery that so often repels the general reader from present-day writings on psychology. A few terms not in common use had perforce to be used freely throughout the book, but each of these was invented in order to name some idea essential to the development of the subject, and is fully explained when it first occurs.

I wish especially to thank Professor Spearman, not only for the inspiration I have drawn from his work, but also for his great kindness in introducing this book. To several helpers I owe thanks, which I cordially offer them here, for reading parts of the typescript and the proofs: Mr A. Charles, Mr A. H. Dodd, Mr F. Kettle, and my wife. To Mr Charles, who read all the proofs with critical care, I owe the improvement of several phrases and the removal of some ambiguities. I am glad to acknowledge the kind permission of Dr Ballard to quote some of his tests.

E. R. HAMILTON.

THE ART OF INTERROGATION

CHAPTER I

THE DESCRIPTION OF MIND—SOME GENERAL PRINCIPLES

1. *Introductory*

To understand other people's minds, and to act in accordance with such understanding, are vital concerns of everybody. Not only is our behaviour in daily intercourse with others determined largely by our beliefs as to the nature of their minds, but most of our thinking, the private side of our life, is coloured by meanings derived from our social life. We cannot, in fact, understand our own minds unless we have some understanding of the minds of other people ; nor can we interpret other minds except in terms of experience of our own. The psychologist has a triple task to perform. He must try to see others as he sees himself ; he must try to see others as they see themselves ; and he, like all men, must value the " giftie " to see himself as others see him. Psychology is the science of describing other minds in terms of one's own mind, and one's own in terms of others. No study could well be more important or more fascinating than that of the means by which we seek to estimate and classify the mental qualities of our fellows.

There are many ways in which we seek to obtain knowledge, or to form opinions, of the mental qualities of men. In a task so essential to all men's welfare as the judgment of the nature of their fellows all must have some skill, however crude, however uncertain, however unconsciously acquired. Many people develop, in the course of everyday life, considerable power of judging character and other qualities in an intuitive way ; that is to say, they can make those judgments, but they do not know how they make them. And he is no psychologist in whose estimations of the mental qualities of individuals intuitive judgment does not play a large part. It is the business of the psychologist, however, at once to respect intuition and to suspect it. He, therefore, devises systematic methods of examination to supplement his intuitions. It is with such systematic methods that we are concerned in this book.

2. *Descriptive Terms and Enduring Qualities*

In order that we may compare individuals with respect to their mental qualities we must have some system of describing minds, a vocabulary of terms that can be applied to recognizable mental qualities. And these terms must be applicable in the same sense to the minds of all the individuals whom we wish to compare with one another. If by " memory " we mean something recognizable in the mind of Smith, the term must not be meaningless when applied to the mind of Robinson. If we speak of " intelligence ", we must mean the same kind of thing when we are speaking of Smith's mind as when we are speaking of Robinson's ; and we must mean the same kind of thing when we use the term to describe Smith's skill in mathematics as when we use it to describe his skill in laying a fire. The ideal towards which we must work— and we are always far from attaining it—is a vocabulary by which we can describe the mind of *any* person (given the necessary knowledge of his mental nature), and such that every term has a definite meaning, which is the same in its application to all individuals, at all times, and in all circumstances.

Let us see more clearly what can be meant by the phrase " describing a mind ". What justification is there for talking of " describing a man's mind ", as we have done, as though his " mind " were something he carried about with him, a thing we could look upon and see that it was good—or bad, or indifferent ? Now, this question will lead us, if we let it, into difficulties literally as great as we please. But our present purpose will be served by an answer of a comparatively simple character.

Experience shows that many of the observable attributes of men endure for a considerable time. If a man is described as " clever ", the description is supposed to hold good for many years, although he may be in " good form " one day and in " poor form " another. If we have formed the opinion that a certain man is " good ", we are shocked to find him in jail for embezzlement, for the saint of Monday is not usually the criminal of Tuesday. If Dr Johnson is said to have been hypochondriacal it is because hypochondria was one of his enduring characteristics. The point need not be further laboured. Obviously neither psychology, nor indeed much of human intercourse, would be possible were it not for the fact that many qualities of human beings are permanent or semi-permanent. Upon this fact is dependent, in particular, the value of all examining and testing of men. For, we must suppose, in classifying or selecting individuals for any purpose, that the classification obtained at the time of the test will continue, for some time at least, to hold good.

Common sense recognizes some of the exceptions to which the assumption of the permanence of human qualities is subject. It recognizes that a man's efficiency depends partly upon what he has had for dinner, and that efficiency may vary with the state of health from month to month or from year to year. It recognizes that his nervousness may temporarily reduce the effective ability of a good candidate in an examination ; that a keen mind may rust through disuse ; that experience of an unusual kind may sometimes work sudden and great changes in a man, so that his emotional nature may be transformed into something that would have been quite strange to him the day before. Such catastrophic transformations are, however, rare, and variations of efficiency and character generally take place about a fairly stable norm.

Turning now to the metaphor of "possessing a mind", we may justify it by pointing to the permanence or semi-permanence of human qualities. Since an individual shows certain uniformities in his behaviour, certain characteristic degrees of skill, certain tendencies to action, certain emotional traits, and so on, it is convenient to think of these constancies as manifestations of an enduring something, and that something is what, in this chapter, we have been calling a "mind". This is the sense in which we shall generally use the term "mind" in this book. When we speak of "mental qualities" we shall not usually mean what a man observes by introspection, his feelings, his images, his willings and knowings ; we shall refer rather to the fact that the man is *liable to have* such and such experiences or to display such and such behaviour. We shall think of "mental qualities" as qualities in virtue of which he thinks and feels and desires in certain ways. But the phrase "qualities in virtue of which he thinks . . . in certain ways", is a figure of speech ; all that we actually know is that he *does* think, feel, desire, in certain ways at various times.

These more or less enduring mental qualities, often called " dispositions ", do not necessarily exist, and in any case we have no notion of their nature ; to speak of them as " traces " or as " deposits ", as some psychologists have done, or (still worse) to refer to them as " neurograms ", as others have done, is to make a gratuitous and (as far as the point of view adopted in this book is concerned) an unnecessary hypothesis. When we say that a certain disposition " exists in a man's mind " we mean no more than that he is likely to act or think in a certain way. To say that dispositions exist, is simply to say in other words that present behaviour is in part determined by the history of the individual, including what he inherits from his parents. Instead of saying that the Speaker of the House of Commons will recognize Big Ben next time he sees it, we may say—because it happens to suit our scheme of psychological description—that he has a disposition (more accurately, a " cognitive disposition ") corresponding to Big Ben. Instead of saying that Jones is frequently in a bad temper we say, even in ordinary speech, that he has an " irascible disposition ".

3. *Modes of Description*

In this book we shall be mainly concerned with the task of assessing and describing the more or less enduring characteristics of individuals. But there are various kinds of psychological description. We may describe mental processes as we observe them going on in our own minds (to use the everyday metaphor). Or, we may observe the behaviour of other people or of animals, and describe such behaviour in purely physical terms. Again, we may describe the *behaviour* of man or animal in the sort of terms we use in the description of *mental processes*. Or, when other people make written or spoken signs to us, we may be able to describe, not only the mere behaviour of writing or speaking, but the mental processes we regard as indicated by those signs. And finally, there is the kind of description already referred to ; that namely, of the dispositional nature of an individual—his knowledge, skill, tendencies, abilities and capacities.

With the description of mental processes, with the interpretation of signs, and with dispositional descriptions we need not deal here. A good illustration of the different modes of describing behaviour is provided by Thorndike's well-known experiments on cats. We will describe in two ways what happens in those experiments. A cat, which has had nothing to eat for some time, is placed inside a cage. If a certain string is pulled, or a button struck, inside the cage, the door of the cage will open. A piece of fish is placed outside the cage, beyond the reach of the cat. The cat is found to run about in an apparently haphazard fashion, until in due course it operates the string or button which releases it. When this experiment is repeated many times the animal takes less and less time to escape, finally escaping almost immediately it is placed inside the cage. Here is a description in purely physical terms. Let the reader now contrast this account with the following. A hungry cat, placed in a cage, outside which is placed a piece of fish within sight and smell of the cat, shows signs of great impatience and rushes about excitedly but without any definite plan of action. In the course of these random, or apparently random, movements, the cat will strike the releasing mechanism, probably by accident, and so satisfy its desire to reach the fish. If the cat is placed again and again in the same cage, it will in course of time learn how to get out, and will then escape as soon as it is placed in the cage. This is quite a different kind of description. The terms " hungry ", " sight ", " smell ", " impatience ", " desire ", " learn ", are mental terms ; and most people would regard the second as the truer kind of description. Why they would do so, is an interesting psychological problem.

Let us consider now more particularly the description of the enduring characteristics of individuals : their abilities, capacities, tendencies, beliefs, prejudices, and so forth. In what ways do we obtain the data necessary for describing such qualities ? We may obtain such data by observation of the ways in which men act in their everyday life. Or, the works produced by men, their books or pictures, the bridges or railways they make, the battles they win or lose, may be interpreted as signifying the possession of such and such mental qualities. Again, by subjecting men to systematic tests and examinations, we can try to compare them with one another with respect to specified qualities, their powers of memorizing, their abilities in mathematics, the readiness with which they can perceive relations, or certain kinds of relations, between different things. Each of these methods of obtaining information has its particular merit. Thus, the kind of knowledge we gain of our intimate friends through constant intercourse with them will often enable us to predict with high probability their action in given circumstances, and to do so with more accuracy than we could if we had to rely solely upon the results obtained by subjecting them to a series of psychological tests. Much of our knowledge of acquaintances, however, is obtained intuitively, and is therefore peculiarly liable to bias. A psychological test may be the most dependable means of ascertaining the degree in which an individual possesses a particular mental quality, such as power of visual memory, of discrimination between the pitches of musical notes, or of dealing with problems of a particular kind. On the other hand, men, in the works they spontaneously produce, give us information about their minds that frequently can be obtained neither through personal acquaintance nor by systematic testing.

4. *The Differences between Individuals*

Psychology is possible because all men are alike, and worth while because all men are different. The stress in orthodox psychology used to be upon the resemblances between human beings, mental qualities being discussed in the abstract rather than in the forms they assumed in particular individuals. Actually what the early psychologist did was to confine his attention mainly to his own mind, and then assume that the introspective description he made would apply equally well to the mind of anybody else. And that assumption had this much truth in it : namely, that general psychological concepts, to which definite names could be given, must, if they are valid, be applicable to all minds. But, that we can describe the features of the human face in general terms, does not imply that all human faces are alike !

Psychology became at once more interesting, more useful and more scientific when it began to concern itself with the study of *the ways in which individuals differ from one another*. The old " general psychology " bears to the " psychology of individual differences " a relation in some respects analogous to that between formal grammar and literature. Grammar is possible in so far as there are principles common to all speech ; but literature draws its life from the infinite varieties of speech that are possible. The kind of description we now aim at is a concrete description of the mental qualities of particular individuals, but in doing this we are actuated by the motives of comparing individuals and of seeking laws of mental action that will apply to all individuals alike. And in leaving the old kind of general psychology behind us we have not, of course, relinquished general psychological terms. The vocabulary in terms of which we describe the mind of Smith will be used also to describe the mind of Jones.

There are several ways of comparing the minds of individuals. These ways fall into two roughly distinguishable classes, according to the type of description of mind upon which we base the comparison. Consider first another kind of comparison, *e.g.*, that between two pictures. We may express our judgment of comparison between two pictures by simply saying that one is more pleasing, or has more merit than the other " on the whole ". Or, we may compare the pictures with respect to various qualities, each quality being considered separately : colour, line, design, and so on. Now, in judging a picture " as a whole " we necessarily judge it from some definite point of view—the pleasure it gives, or its æsthetic merit ; we are in that sense judging a single quality of the picture. But in forming such a judgment we must take cognizance, perhaps subconsciously, of the separate qualities (line, colour, etc.) of the picture. Our judgment of the picture as a whole is not, however, simply the sum of the separate judgments (which we need not necessarily express in words) of the various qualities ; nor, indeed, is it the total of those judgments *plus* a further judgment. If, however, we try to make a detailed comparison between two pictures we are sure to make an analysis of their qualities and then compare them with respect to these qualities ; but this analytical comparison is never exhaustive. Similarly, if we wish to make a detailed comparison between the minds of two individuals, we shall be driven to comparing them with respect to particular mental qualities—their intelligence, suggestibility, powers of appreciating music, irascibility, and so on ; and this is what we try to do by means of mental tests. But it is certainly as true of psychological comparison as it is of comparing pictures, that such an analytical comparison does not tell the whole story of the ways in which the individuals differ from one another. In fact, when you have compared Smith's intelligence with that of Jones, and Smith's irascibility with Jones's, and so on throughout the gamut of mental qualities, you have still got to compare *Smith* with *Jones*.

Mental tests are concerned solely with the analytical comparison between individuals : by means of tests we compare individuals with respect to one mental quality at a time ; but a man's expressive product, such as the book he writes or the picture he paints, may give us insight into that balance or synthesis of mental qualities that lends the man his distinctive individuality, insight that no amount of psychological testing would ever afford us.

The question whether there is a sense in which a man's mind may, like a picture, be judged or valued " as a whole ", is one for philosophy rather than psychology. But the distinction between analytical and synthetic judgment is one that will recur frequently in these pages, and it may well receive further illustration at this point.

If we want to ascertain whether Smith or Jones is the better chess player we may satisfy ourselves by getting them to play a number of games together and to solve a number of problems which we have designed as specially searching. In this way we obtain data for a comparison of their total abilities in chess. But a fuller description of their individual differences in the matter of chess-playing would have to indicate that Smith, who is usually beaten by Jones, has his good points, in some of which he is very much superior to Jones. This is the analytical kind of description. Similarly, if we want to know which of two men is the best all-round mathematician, we may set them papers in the various branches of mathematics and base our decision upon the total marks. But if we want to make a complete comparison between the mathematical abilities of the two men, we must break up mathematical skill into components (which need not necessarily correspond to the conventional branches — algebra, geometry, etc.), and make each component the subject of a separate comparison.

Before we leave this preliminary account of the comparison of individuals mention should be made of another point. In any full comparison of the minds of Smith and Jones there will be reference to the degrees in which they respectively appear to possess various mental qualities : intelligence, suggestibility, constancy or fickleness of motives, and so on. But we must also consider the *relations* between these mental qualities in each individual. For, the important thing in the comparison between these two men may be that, whilst Smith's intelligence is far greater than that of Jones, Jones, having great constancy of purpose, makes so much better use of his intelligence that he is, on the whole, the more effective person of the two, and one more likely to succeed in what he undertakes to do. Analytical comparison of individuals needs always to be supplemented by such consideration of the inter-relations between their mental qualities.

A similar proviso is necessary when we turn from the consideration of enduring mental qualities to that of mental processes. The attempt to analyse mental processes into kinds—such as emotions, willings and knowings —especially when it is described as an attempt to analyse mind into parts, is often decried as a falsification of the facts of mental life. A mind broken up, it is said, is no longer a mind. But indeed analysis and abstraction are unavoidable in psychology. It is true that the various mental processes that receive separate names in our analysis are, in the living mind, organically united, or, we had better say, that a " process " is always but one aspect of a whole experience. But, although we may employ one system of psychological categories or another, we are bound, having chosen our system, to consider separately each of those categories. Thus we consider emotion and cognition separately. But we atone for this unavoidable sin by further considering what we describe as " the interaction between emotion and cognition ".

5. *Theoretical and Practical Aims*

Psychology, once but a modest branch of philosophy, has distinguished itself in recent years by the number and variety of its applications to problems of practical life. Its range now extends from philosophy to bricklaying. But the applications always have a theoretical as well as a practical interest. Mental tests, for example (whether they be designed to single out the men most likely to become good rifle shots, or to gauge the capacity of girls for dressmaking, or to select mentally defective children for treatment in special schools), not only serve their various practical purposes, but also contribute to the general theory of psychology. Indeed, the distinction between theoretical and practical aims is often very indefinite. Any statement of the kinds and degrees of an individual's mental qualities, whether made in an account of the psychology of bricklaying or in one of the psychology of philosophical thinking, implies a certain scheme of psychological description, and such a scheme in its turn implies some hypothesis of the nature of mental action.

6. *Ambiguity of Terms*

This dependence of the psychologist's vocabulary of descriptive terms upon his knowledge of, and theories concerning, mental action is one of those obvious things that we seem to be always recognizing and never understanding. The part played by words in his science presents perhaps the most difficult and fundamental of the problems with which the psychologist is faced, and it would be impertinence to make any approach to the problem that might suggest that we intended attacking it here. Nevertheless our outline of the principles of psychological description would have serious gaps if nothing whatever were said about the meanings of terms.

It would be pedantic to demand that any word should always carry the same meaning, and it would be impossible to comply with the demand. Psychological terms must change their meaning as our knowledge increases, and most of them must play more than one part. We can never tie a word down to one narrow meaning and be sure that it will behave itself and mean just that one thing in all contexts, at all times, to all people. We cannot reach final and perfect definition of words, and it would perhaps be the end of literature if we could ; but in psychology we must always be acting as though our aim was to reach such definition.

If we say that a child who suffers from night fears has a " strong imagination ", and we say the same of an engineer or a poet, we know quite well that the psychological import of the term " imagination " is quite different in the three cases. There is no confusion of thought in this triple use of the term " imagination ", though there is perhaps a poverty of language. But confusion arises when we forget how different may be the psychological import of a word in different contexts, or as used by different people. Thus if what one man means by " intelligence " is " capacity to profit by experience ", and what another man means by the same word is " all-round mental efficiency ", it is clear that they cannot profitably use the word in conversation with one another.

We have to use language in psychology and we have to pay for it by constant risk of error. There are two principal ways in which we may incur this risk. " Memory " well illustrates this. We may use the same word at different times with different meanings. Thus, by " memory " may be meant the *process* of recalling past experiences ; or the *power* of long delayed recall ; or the power of " memorizing " measured by the accuracy of immediate recall ; or (in common speech) the fact recalled : and these are all very different meanings. This kind of ambiguity is often removed by the context in which the word occurs. The second kind of ambiguity referred to above is more subtle. Even if we confine the word " memory " to the meaning " power of recall " we are still liable to the following kind of error. We are still tempted to believe that recall of one kind of material is psychologically the same process as recall of another kind of material : that a good memory for what is seen operates through the same causes, and therefore implies, a good memory for what is heard ; that a good memory for faces implies also a good memory for poetry ; that memory, in fact, is a quite general mental power, equally applicable to all kinds of materials. The plain man does not always make this mistake ; he asserts that he has a good memory for faces whilst making no pretence of being able to remember the gist of the books he reads. But he asserts that so and so has a " good memory ", without realizing that such a term has not got the meaning he implies, unless excellence in one kind of memory always goes with excellence in all other kinds.

Whilst the plain man may sometimes overlook the existence of different kinds of memory, the psychologist finds a considerable problem in the very existence of those " kinds ". For, he is driven to inquire whether the common element in all kinds of memory is a merely logical one (is the fact, namely, that all memory involves reference to past experiences), or whether there is a psychological element common to all kinds of memory.

In the case also of a term such as " judgment ", the existence of the general term is apt to blind us, if we are not watching our psychological paces, to the fact that there may be judgment of more than one kind. Thus, using the word " judge " in the popular sense of " one who discriminates between merits ", we may say that a man may be a good judge of pictures but a poor judge of melodies, a good judge of horses but a poor judge of men. Here again, the plain man realizes that this lack of cor- relation between different " kinds " of judgment exists. But he does not realize the considerable theoretical problem raised by our use of a common term to cover such a variety of mental processes or operations. All acts of judgment have something in common which leads us to call them by the same name. But of what nature must that " something in common " between the different species of a psychological genus be in order that we may legitimately regard them as species of the same genus ?

We must expect to find some differences in the applica-

bility of any given psychological term to different
individuals. This is another kind of ambiguity that
psychological terms are heir to. Let us illustrate this
by examples. Confronted by a mind that bore no
resemblance to the human, our psychology would break
down at the task of describing it. We need not wait for
a Martian to visit us before a concrete illustration of this
point is at hand. The psychologist in describing the
mind of an ape uses the same terms (intelligence, fear,
sympathy, and so forth) as he uses to describe the human
mind. The biological kinship between man and ape is
so close that it seems reasonable to assume a close
resemblance, in some respects, between the mind of the
ape and that of man. Even so, we can easily suppose the
resemblance to be stronger than it is. But when the
psychologist turns his attention to insects and animals
of low degree he feels much less confidence in his vocabulary. The " fear " of an insect is probably so different
from the emotion so called in man and the higher animals
that the very use of the word as applied to the insect is
at best a makeshift. The difference so obvious here
exists, but in far less degree, as between different men.
My emotions of fear are in some respects peculiar to me,
but they are the subject-matter of psychology only to the
extent to which they resemble the emotion that goes by
the same name in other men.

7. *The Principle of Indication*

The facts upon which we base our psychological
description of an individual are his actions, his sayings,
his works, his responses to situations of various kinds.
We judge the man by what he does or produces, either as
responses to our tests or as responses to the test of life

itself. The latter is the method of the biographer, and is no concern of this book ; the former is the method of the examiner and the experimental psychologist.

Having subjected an individual to some kind of examination or psychological test, we ask : What does his performance in the test tell us about this individual ? And to this question there is at once available an obvious and generally useless answer : the answer, namely, that at the time of the test he was able to produce these particular responses. But since the qualities in virtue of which he made those responses may usually be supposed to endure for some time (cp. Section 2), we should usually add without hesitation that the individual could again, apart from memory of his first attempt, make the same responses to the test. That is to say, we should generally regard his test performance as indicating a more or less enduring ability to answer this particular test with a certain degree of success. But as a rule we should also feel justified in concluding that his performance indicated his ability to deal with tests similar to, but not identical with, the test we have applied to him. Thus, if our test required him to reproduce from memory a simple design which had been shown to him for a short interval, we should regard the success with which he performed this task as indicating with high probability the success with which he could reproduce a somewhat *different* design which was shown to him for the same length of time. But we might make (of course, with greater risk of error) a still wider inference from our test results ; we might infer, not only that the individual had such and such a power of reproducing designs in general, but also that he would probably display ability of a certain degree in describing from memory the appearance and arrangement of various objects that lay on a table which he was

B

allowed to observe for an interval. Indeed, the design-reproduction test, especially if it was repeated many times with various designs, might conceivably be justly regarded as indicating the individual's general power of visual memory. This would be an instance of what is in fact a general rule : the rule, namely, that *an individual's performance in a given test usually tells us a good deal more about the individual than just the mere fact that he can answer that particular test with such and such a degree of success.*

Any number of instances of this rule may be found. When a man is subjected to a test of " intelligence ", we infer, not only that he has displayed a certain degree of intelligence in the particular situation of the test, but that his performance gives some indication of the intelligence he can bring to bear upon situations that differ from the test-situation. On the basis of a candidate's examination essay we try to judge, not only his power of writing essays on the particular theme set, but also his power of writing in general ; not that only, but also his ability in the subject of the examination ; and much else. Indeed it is obvious that examinations and psychological tests would have but little significance if we could only take the results at, so to speak, their face value. We must always infer that the test results are significant of something beyond themselves, that they indicate certain qualities which they do not directly test. I propose to refer to this fact as the " principle of wider indication ", or, more briefly, as the " principle of indication ".

There seem to be two main reasons for our belief in the principle of indication. The first reason is the fact that there is some degree of uniformity in the actions of individuals. Psychology has to make an assumption corresponding to the physicist's assumption of the uniformity of nature ; but this assumption, though it is a *sine qua non* of a science of psychology, is much more likely to be misapplied in psychology than in physical science. We assume then that performance in a test indicates at least an ability, which will endure for some time, to deal with situations of the kind presented in the test. The second fact underlying the principle of indication is the evident one that there are elements common to different kinds of activity, different kinds of experience, and different kinds of behaviour. When we notice the ease with which a person learns to play tennis, we conclude that he will probably not find great difficulty in learning badminton, for some of the factors of skill in tennis are also factors of skill in badminton. But the indication of a given performance may have various degrees of definiteness.   Can we conclude, for example, from the fact that Smith beats Jones in jigsaw puzzles that he is likely to beat Jones in wire puzzles or in a game of chess ?   Or, if neither man knows the game of chess, may we conclude, from the fact that Smith is greatly superior to Jones in mathematics, that he is likely to learn chess with greater ease than is possible for Jones ?   This last question can only be answered (*i.e.*, the width of the indication of a mathematical test can only be ascertained) by experiment.

We are constantly using this " principle of indication " in our everyday interpretations of men's actions. We are constantly regarding particular actions as having a significance beyond the fact that the individual can do those particular things. The man who performs several remarkable feats at billiards can almost certainly, we believe, perform others. The man who constructs a well-knit argument about one philosophical topic can almost certainly, we believe, reason well about some other philosophical topics.   If we are listening to a conversation, or watching the gambols of our dog on a walk, or testing the intelligence of deaf-mutes in our laboratory, we are interested in what we observe in each case chiefly because of its wider indication. We regard it as indicating certain mental processes taking place at the time in man or dog ; we may regard it as indicating certain probabilities as to future action of the individual, as indicating, that is to say, certain enduring characteristics of the individual. The dog's gambols denote a healthy and a happy dog ; the dog's solution of a problem, such as that of lifting a door-latch, indicates a probability that the dog will be able to solve other problems : we are very ready, if he is our own dog, to regard the act as betokening " intelligence ", a general power of performing acts for which he has not been trained. Our friend's witty sayings raise the hope and encourage the belief that he will continue to make other witty remarks. If some of the factors upon which wit may appear to depend—such as, clearness of thought, or the power to observe resemblances, which most people would not notice, between things—may operate in other ways than in the production of wit, then his wittiness has some power of indication of the individual's power to act in those other ways. Again, if a candidate reaches a certain level in an academic examination we make a Civil Servant of him. We do not want him to translate Latin or to solve mathematical problems in his administrative capacity, but we regard ability in Latin and mathematics as " indicative " of other qualities that *will* operate in the performance of the Civil Servant's duties. At this point we begin to see the need for caution in the application of the principle of indication. For, it is surely conceivable that the academic examination may *not* indicate abilities outside the sphere of the examination. The question as to how much difference, and what kind of difference, there can be between one kind of activity and another kind, in order that performance in the first kind shall be " indicative " of power to perform in the second, is a very fundamental question, to which we shall return in the next chapter.

8. *Recapitulation*

The possibility of describing minds rests upon two main supports : the resemblance between different human beings, which enables us, by the process of abstraction, to create a vocabulary of descriptive terms applicable to the minds of all men ; and the fact that most qualities of an individual are permanent or semi-permanent, a fact which gives our descriptions their chief value. We pointed out that in order to make a full psychological comparison between individuals it was in general necessary to analyse their mental qualities and make a separate comparison with respect to each quality. But the separate description of each of an individual's mental qualities does not provide us with a complete description of the individual : it is also necessary to consider the interrelation between the various qualities. We proceeded to consider the errors to which we may be led by the necessity of using language in psychology, suggesting that a considerable problem was raised by the unavoidable use of terms such as " memory ", " judgment ", etc., each of which might cover mental processes or powers of various kinds. The theoretical problem of the nature of general terms we passed by, but the practical consequences of the fact that such general terms as "memory", etc., do not always denote a unitary mental power, were mentioned—that, for example, we could not suppose that good memory for one kind of material necessarily implied good memory for another kind. On the other hand, it was then pointed out that we were constantly and necessarily using observed mental qualities as the basis of inferences, constantly regarding a man's behaviour in one kind of situation, the mode of operation of his mind upon one kind of material, as significant of his power to react to other kinds of situation or material : the possibility of doing this was called the " principle of indication ".

Some of the ways in which we gain information about other minds were mentioned.   We form opinions about the mental qualities of men by observing the ways in which they act, the things they say and do ; some of our opinions are formed intuitively, whilst others are the result of deliberate attempts to assess and describe the minds of men.   Of the deliberate modes of observation there are two broadly distinguishable classes : on the one hand, observation of the responses men make, and the works they produce, in the ordinary course of their lives ; on the other hand, observation of their reactions to situations specially designed to test their qualities.   Our theme in this book is the last-named method.   As the method generally consists in requiring individuals to answer questions, and as the applying of any test, whatever its form, is always tantamount to asking a particular question concerning the mind of the testee, we may well give this method of investigation the name that stands on our title-page : The Art of Interrogation.

CHAPTER II

THE WAY OF MENTAL TESTS

1. *Introductory*

THE way with which we are concerned in this and the ensuing chapters of obtaining information about the kinds and degrees of men's mental qualities consists in the systematic observation of their reactions to specially designed situations. Any situation might be called a " mental test " when we study and compare the reactions of people to it, and we shall sometimes use the term " mental test " in this very broad sense. In recent years, however, the term has acquired a highly specific meaning, with which the reader is doubtless familiar ; it generally refers to a test designed primarily with a view to reliably comparing individuals with respect to some given mental quality, such as "intelligence", power of voluntary attention, specific skills or aptitudes, power of perceiving relations between things, and so on.

Nothing in the history of psychology is more remarkable than the success with which "mental tests " (in the narrower sense of the term, to which reference has just been made) have been employed by some psychologists ; nothing more lamentable than the triviality to which others have been led by the same methods. The far-reaching significance of the more judicious applications of mental tests, and the dangerous popularity of the more futile, alike call for a review of the assumptions that underlie their use.

2. *Expression and Interpretation*

The possibility of mental testing rests upon the occurrence of *significant behaviour* and *expressive signs*. In a truly wonderful way we are able to interpret the behaviour and the expressions of other people in mental terms : we are able, that is to say, on hearing a man speak or seeing him act, to think, with greater or less accuracy according to circumstances, of the mental processes he is experiencing, of his thoughts, his motives and feelings.   How the communication of experience by means of language and other signs is possible is a mystery which we are not here called upon to probe. Our humbler purpose will be served by a few examples of the interpretation of behaviour or of signs.

A man may describe his own mental processes. Such a description is an expressive product. But what it directly expresses is the man's attempt at introspection, and he may be able to introspect well or ill.   Introspective reports have great value as sources of psychological data, but their utility is restricted in several ways. First, introspection is a difficult process which different people may practise with various degrees of competence. Secondly, although we may often have sufficient reason for rejecting a person's report as unreliable, we cannot directly check the validity of a given report. Thirdly, introspection can only tell us directly about *mental processes ;* it usually tells us little about dispositions or tendencies.   The chief use of introspective reports for the mental tester is that of checking the assumption he is bound to make that the solution of a given test is reached by such and such a kind of mental process.   If he learns from the introspective reports of testees that some of them have correctly answered a test by one kind of mental process, whilst others have correctly answered the same test by another kind of process, then he will have to reject that test as an ambiguous one.

As an example of significant behaviour we may take that of a man whom we observe running away from a tiger. This event could be described in purely geometrical terms, just as we might describe the relative motion of two billiard balls. The physicist, in order to describe the interaction between the billiard balls, introduces unobservable things, such as force, energy, and momentum. In describing the man and the tiger we introduce the hypothesis that they are experiencing certain mental processes : the man is frightened and wishes to escape ; he knows something about the manners, or lack of manners, of tigers ; the tiger is hungry and desires to eat the man. In these mental interpretations we may be wrong. We should probably be wrong in supposing the man to be frightened of the tiger if the event took place in a circus ; but then if we observed it in a circus we should very likely not suppose that fear had anything to do with the man's running away. The interpretation we put upon behaviour, then, depends not only upon the character of the behaviour, but also upon the circumstances in which it is observed—a fact of great importance in the theory of mental testing.

All behaviour is significant, in the sense that, observing the behaviour, *we infer more than just that such and such behaviour is taking place.* But, as we have just seen, the same action on the part of a man may signify different things according to circumstances. If we observe a man running rapidly along a street we may generally assume that he is experiencing certain muscular sensations, unless it happens that he is running in his sleep or is otherwise unconscious of what he is doing. If a tiger or a policeman is observed running after the man, the man's behaviour at once takes on a more specific psychological significance : we infer that he is probably feeling some degree of fear or anxiety, and that he is looking for a way of escape—at least in the sense that, as soon as an opportunity for escape presents itself, it is more likely to be perceived by the man than if he were running merely for exercise.   If the man is discovered to be merely an actor in one of those popular cinema dramas, whose aim is to give people the thrill of being chased without the physical exertion of running or the possible evil consequences of being caught, we shall have been quite wrong in our inference as to the nature of his mental processes.   He who runs may do many things—may think in so many different ways, feel such diverse emotions, be intent upon carrying out so many kinds of purpose, that the psychological implication of the mere act of running is very ambiguous.

Compare now the running man with a man working some kind of mental test.   The man is presented with a wire puzzle and instructed to separate the interlocked pieces.[1]   What is generally observed in such an experiment, and what we find ourselves doing when we try such a puzzle, is that for a while the pieces are pulled about in what seems like a random way ;   the observer sees no relation between the procedure and the procedure required to solve the puzzle.   But presently (and with some people from the first) behaviour is observed which we regard as having a psychological significance quite different from that of the random manipulations.   The speed of manipulation is slackened, pieces are moved slowly round about certain relative positions, the movements show a more

[1] See the account of H. A. Ruger's experiments with wire puzzles in *The Growth of the Mind*, by K. Koffka, pp. 174-9.   International Library of Psychology, 1924.

definite relation to the shapes of the pieces. We infer that the testee is exploring the parts of the puzzle, that his explorations are guided by his perceptions of the relations between the parts and by his knowledge of what he is trying to accomplish. If he keeps the pieces for some time in a certain relative position, and slowly moves them about that position, we infer that he thinks he is probably on the right tack. And finally, when the pieces come apart, we suppose that the testee understands as we do why they come apart. If, moreover, he holds the pieces for a while together in the position in which they can be separated, we feel confident in inferring that he is trying to register that position in memory in order that he may solve the puzzle without hesitation when he next tries it.

Now it is clear that, quite apart from any introspective report the man may give us, it is much easier to give an account of the cognitive processes the man is probably experiencing when he solves the wire puzzle than it is to describe his mental processes when we merely observe him running down a street. It is also clear, and this is the important point, that if we set a number of people to solve the same wire puzzle, the cognitive processes associated with any particular manipulation of the pieces will probably be much the same in the mind of any one of the people as in that of any other. This is especially true of the manipulations they make when they are on the verge of the solution. Anybody solving the puzzle, otherwise than by accident, would have to understand certain relations between the pieces; the tester knows what those relations are, and he can therefore interpret success in the puzzle as betokening at least the power of understanding such relations. Interpretation, then, of the behaviour of people solving a wire puzzle may be made with some confidence, though not without risk of error. We are able to make several assumptions which facilitate the interpretation : we know that all the people are aiming at the same end ; we know that they all have knowledge of the simple spatial relations between things (such as that a protuberance on one piece of the puzzle can, if the arrangements of the other parts of the puzzle permit, be passed through a nick on another piece of the puzzle) ; we know that when they think they are on the way to the solution they will more closely observe the relative positions of the pieces. Nevertheless, we must recognize that here it is no more true than it was in the case of the running man that a particular kind of behaviour *necessarily* indicates one kind of mental process, and that one only. For example, if the only part of the man's behaviour that we witnessed was the final separation of the pieces, we should have no means of knowing whether he had reached that result by reasoning or by accident, or by a mixture of the two. Moreover, when we observe the man making tentative manipulations in the early stages of the solution, we cannot judge from the observed movements alone what degree of insight into the conditions of the problem the man is experiencing.

The wire puzzle is not a typical " mental test," but it clearly illustrates some of the conditions of testing and some of the problems we have to face in the design of tests. The important qualities of the puzzle, considered as a test, are the following. First, the puzzle, considered as a whole, presents the *same problem* to all the individuals we are testing. They all know exactly what they must try to do, so that, however diverse the procedures different individuals may adopt, we know that they are all carried out with the same final aim in view. This is an essential condition of any mental test, but, as we shall see later, it is a condition that we cannot always secure so easily as we can in the case of the wire puzzle. Secondly, what follows from the first condition, the problem to be solved is perfectly definite and admits of only one correct answer : apart from the fact that the pieces will be separable if placed in any relative position between certain narrow limits, a fact which causes no confusion, we know when an individual has solved the puzzle, and *he* knows also. It is usually the aim of the mental tester to devise tests which the testee either passes or fails, and in which he cannot be half right ; but mental testers do not always secure this condition in their tests ; and a question in an ordinary examination paper (in history, for example) may admit of answers of many degrees of " correctness ". Thirdly, the puzzle illustrates some of the problems of the interpretation of individuals' performances. Thus, it raises the problem of " difficulty." Some individuals will solve the problem more quickly than others : can we conclude that its solution was easier for them than for their slower competitors ? We can draw that conclusion to the extent to which they were not aided by lucky manipulations. Shall we regard the times taken by various individuals to solve the puzzle as indicating inversely their relative abilities to solve this kind of puzzle ? We can make no inference as to ability, unless the effects of chance upon the individuals' performances are eliminated. The greatest enemy of chance in mental testing is multiplication of tests. Let us, then, set our testees several different wire puzzles. Shall we now regard the ability of an individual in wire puzzles as indicated by the speed with which on the average he solves them ? Or, shall we not rather consider the *complexity* of the puzzles as determining the ability required to solve them, so that, the puzzles having been arranged in a scale according to their objective (geo-metrical) complexity, the ability of an individual is indicated by the position he can reach in that scale ? Can we be sure, however, that the objective complexity of a puzzle is the sole determinant of the difficulty the testee feels in his endeavour to solve it ?   Practice in this kind of puzzle may improve performance, and some testees may be practised whilst others are not.   Moreover, it is clear that the most able individuals will *feel less difficulty* in the task than do the less able.

The wire puzzle, having raised for us a number of difficult problems, may now be allowed to retire from these pages.   Some of these problems we shall consider in this chapter, others in the next.

Suppose now that, instead of giving a man a wire puzzle to solve, we set him what is commonly called an " intelligence test ".   Some of these tests, especially those intended for use with individuals of low-grade mentality, require the testee to manipulate objects.[1]   These belong to the same general class as the wire puzzle and raise no further problems that we wish to consider here.   But most " intelligence tests " demand, not the manipulation of apparatus, but written or spoken responses.   Of this kind are most of the tests in the Binet-Simon series, whilst " Group Tests ", which are applied to many individuals simultaneously, have of necessity to depend upon the written response.   The testee expresses his answers simply by making certain marks on paper—certain crosses and strokes, certain words or numbers—underlining words, and so on.   Here, as in the case of an ordinary written examination, the actual overt behaviour of the man, his actual writing or making of other marks, is of no con-

[1] *E.g.*, the Porteous Maze Tests, the Koh Block-Design Test, and the Healy Formboard Test.

sequence in the interpretation of the test (unless, as may
be the case in an ordinary examination, the slowness with
which the candidate can manipulate a pen is a real
hindrance to him; but this is a trivial point). The
essential difference between the wire puzzle and the
intelligence test lies in the fact that the nature of the
signs to be interpreted is different. With the puzzle
the sign was a form of behaviour, in the intelligence test
the sign is usually some kind of verbal expression. Thus,
in the intelligence test the individual might be asked to
underline the word in the brackets that best completes
the following " analogy " :

Inquiry is to *Curiosity* as *Eating* is to—
(*Drinking, Hunger, Interest, Sleep*).[1]

The essential similarity between the wire puzzle and
the intelligence test lies in the facts that in both there
is one correct answer and only one, and that, provided
that we can be sure that the testee has not solved the
puzzle or the test by chance, we can in both infer with
great confidence the kind of mental process by which
he arrived at the result. In order that he may, without
the aid of chance, solve the " analogy " correctly, it is
necessary that the testee shall see that the relation of
effect to cause, which holds between *Inquiry* and *Curiosity*,
also holds between *Eating* and *Hunger*, but not between
Eating and *Drinking*, or between *Eating* and either
Interest or *Sleep*.[2]

[1] Quoted from *A Measure of " Intelligence "*, by C. Spearman (1925).
[2] This " analogy ", like most that have been devised, is to some
extent *loose*, in that *Eating* may sometimes be due, for example, to
Interest (as when we sample a food although we are not hungry) ; but
the most frequent cause of *Eating* is *Hunger*; the " intelligent " person
would realize this looseness of the analogy, whilst at the same time
realizing that the answer he was expected to give was *Hunger*.

The ideal test would have to satisfy several conditions, of which the only one we need mention here is this : the response made by any individual must have an unambiguous significance. Knowing that a given individual has correctly answered our test, we must be at once able to infer that he possesses the quality whose presence the test is intended to indicate ; knowing that he has failed in the test we must know without doubt that he lacks that quality.

3. *Clearness of Indication*

Every act of a man is psychologically significant, but some acts are more readily interpretable than others. The mental tester subjects individuals to situations which evoke, or which he hopes will evoke, responses which have a fairly definite indication. In order that he may know what a given test indicates he has to analyse the process of solution as it takes place in his own mind. He has then to seek for other possible mental processes by which the test might be solved. Suppose, for instance, to quote the " analogy " form of test again, that the following test is put :

Ink is to *Black* as *Snow* is to—
(*White, Ice, Write, Fall*).

Here there is indeed only one correct answer, but it may be reached by one or the other of two distinct mental processes. It may be reached by perceiving that the relation of *Ink* to *Black* is that of a thing to one of its attributes, and that *Snow* has that relation to *White :* or it may be reached without this perception of a relation, but simply through the operation of the association of *Snow* with *White*. The test is therefore unacceptable, since we have no means of knowing which of the two methods has been employed by any particular testee who gives the correct answer. Every mental test should be subjected by its inventor to as close a scrutiny as possible, in order that he may detect ambiguities of the kind just mentioned, or of a more subtle character. Such analysis of the processes involved in the solution of particular tests has not always been attempted by the makers of tests. Indeed it is possible to devise tests of great variety and much ingenuity without having any clear idea of the processes involved in their solution. *Some* such idea we must have before we can invent a test at all, but our aim should be to invent tests which call for mental processes with which we are tolerably familiar. One way of achieving this is to limit our choice of problems to those which involve only one or two steps in their solution, and that is generally the way of mental tests.

It is not, I think, always necessary, though it is usually advisable, to design tests that shall have only one correct answer. One of the earliest, and in many respects one of the most successful mental tests is the " Completion Test," invented by Ebbinghaus. In a test of that kind which I recently gave to Training College students, the testees were required to put an appropriate word in each of the gaps in the following passage [1] :—

" Once upon a ——— the Prince of Felicitas had ——— to set forth on a ———. It was a late autumn ——— with a few pale stars and a ——— no ——— than the paring of a finger-nail. As he ——— through the purlieus of his city, the white mane of his amber-coloured ——— was ——— that he could clearly see in the dusk of the high streets. His ——— led through a ——— but little known to ———, and he was ——— to find that his

---

[1] From " A Novelist's Allegory ", in *The Inn of Tranquillity*, by John Galsworthy.

C

———, instead of ambling forward with his ——— gentle vigour, stepped carefully from side to side, ———, now and then to curve his ——— and prick his ———, as though at something of fear unseen in the ———."

Now here it is certainly not true that one word and one only can be found for each gap. But in no case was there any doubt as to whether a given answer should be treated as correct or incorrect. Most students completed the first sentence in the form : " Once upon a *time* the Prince of Felicitas had *occasion* to set forth on a *journey* ". Some, however, wrote *determined* in place of *occasion*, and had to be scored as correct. Some put *voyage* in place of *journey*, an answer which is given the lie by the remaining sentences of the passage. The students who in the tests as a whole showed themselves to be less able than the majority frequently completed the third sentence as follows : " As he *rode* through the purlieus of his city, the white mane of his amber-coloured *horse* was *such* that he could clearly see in the dusk of the high streets". The majority of the students wrote *all* in place of *such* in this sentence. The test is defective, not so much because there is doubt as to whether a given answer should be regarded as correct or as wrong, as because the mental process of filling in a gap is so complex that it is hard to know what psychological interpretation to put upon a successful response. There is one direction in which, however, we might seek to justify the test. Without attempting an analysis of the process of solving the test, we may ascertain whether those testees who correctly solve it do in fact possess in high degree the quality that the whole set of tests (of which this Completion Test was but one) is intended to indicate. Suppose, for example, that the tests were intended to indicate average ability (*i.e.*, the average of all the diverse abilities of an individual).

Then, if there is a high degree of correlation between average ability in this sense and ability to solve this Completion Test correctly, the latter may be retained in our set of tests. In that case the psychological interpretation of the Completion Test will depend upon the possibility of putting a *psychological* (as distinct from a merely numerical) interpretation upon the phrase " average of diverse abilities ".

Whilst our task of interpretation of tests is always simplified if we can arrange that they have each only one correct answer, we should unduly cripple ourselves if we excluded all tests which did not tie the testee in this manner. Such a test as the following,[1] for example, would have to be rejected ; yet this test has many virtues. The testee is provided with a diagram consisting of a circle which has a gap at one point in its circumference. This circle represents a field, the gap being the entrance to the field. Supposing that a ball has been lost in the grass, that we do not know from what direction or with what force the ball came, how shall we proceed in order to find the ball as soon as possible ? The testee is instructed to draw with his pencil the path, starting from the entrance, which he would follow in his search. The actual paths chosen by different children are, of course, infinite in variety. Yet it is possible to classify the answers and to say with fair confidence which of them should be regarded as passing the testee and which as failing him. Some children may work their way on a spiral path from the circumference to the centre of the field ; others may follow a wavy path which takes them across and across the field on a series of parallel lines ; others may go straight to the centre of the field and then explore along

---

[1] To be found in the set of tests known as " The Stanford Revision of the Binet-Simon Tests ", by L. Terman.

a series of radii. All these are correct answers, for they indicate that the child realizes that the search must follow some definite plan. The defective child merely makes a single stroke across the circle or produces a scribble which has no design. Here we have a test which is far from the ideal of " one test, one answer ", and a test, moreover, of which the complete analysis would be very complicated. Yet, as one of a series of tests designed as a whole to indicate " general ability ", the test plays its part very well.

Let the reader now observe a significant difference between the test just described (known as the " Ball and Field " test) and the " Analogy " test, of which we have given examples above. In the Ball and Field test the testee is asked to solve a problem of a kind that might well arise in almost the same form in life, whilst " analogies ", in the form in which they appear in mental tests, lead a sequestered life in the psychologist's laboratory. The analogy owes its value and popularity to the relative simplicity of the mental process by which it is solved. Though we can multiply analogy tests indefinitely, they may all be solved by the same general type of mental process. That process is one of the fundamental elements of all thinking ; [1] it is a process which enters into the solution of the Ball and Field test or of any problem whatever. With that process [2] in mind we can devise any number of analogies. We cannot in the same way regard the Ball and Field test as evoking a single specific

[1] The fundamental nature of the Analogy test is revealed in what is unquestionably the most remarkable book that has yet appeared on mental testing : *The Nature of " Intelligence " and the Principles of Cognition*, by C. Spearman (1923).

[2] The process of solving an Analogy has really two parts : the eduction of the appropriate relation between the first two terms of the Analogy ; followed by the " eduction of a correlate ", with respect to the relation so educed, to the third term of the Analogy.

mental process which might also be evoked in a large number of other problems, all of which could be grouped into one class as we can group analogies together.

What might be called the " primary indication " of success in an Analogy test is that the testee has performed the feat of educing a certain relation (usually one of many that might be educed) between the first two terms of the Analogy, and then that of educing a correlate to the third term of the Analogy. What is the primary indication of success in the Ball and Field test ? It might be expressed thus : the testee realized the need for a systematic procedure in the solution of the problem, and he showed such and such realization of spatial relationships in the way in which he planned the procedure. Such an indication, however, carries our analysis very little way ; appreciation of the need for a systematic procedure and appreciation of spatial relations are both psychologically complex experiences. Whilst, therefore, we may well be able to justify this test as an element in a series of tests devised primarily to serve some practical purpose, as an instrument for psychological research the test has serious weakness.

4. *Simplifying the Indication*

In order to simplify the interpretation of test responses the mental tester takes certain precautions. His first concern, though not necessarily his ultimate object, is to be able to infer from an individual's response to any test the mental process by which he solved the test. To this point we have already given some slight consideration. The mental tester tries to devise problems which can be solved by one process of thinking only, or such that the mental processes by which any two individuals solve them have certain essential characteristics in common. Thus one testee solving an Analogy may have an attitude of boredom towards the task, whilst another attacks it with zest ; yet if both solve the test correctly, and the Analogy has been carefully designed, we know at least that each individual educed a certain relation and a certain correlate.

The next concern of the mental tester must be to ensure that if an individual fails to respond correctly to a test, it is because he really lacks the power to do so. This brings us to the important subject of the *Instructions* by which, so to speak, the mental tester sets his stage. If he wants to see whether the testees can solve a certain problem, he must first make clear to them what the problem is. He must initiate them into the rules of the test game. Merely to confront a class of children with the problem [1] :—

> *Handle* is to *Hammer* as *Knob* is to—
> (*Key ? Door ? Shut ? Room ?*),

followed by many others of a like kind, would be to leave some children, *who have the power to solve the Analogies correctly*, uncertain what was the task we wanted them to perform. Some of these children may be confused by the use of the expression " is to ", which hitherto they have met only in arithmetic. All the children might well wonder why four answers were given. The instructions may be very brief, if the test is of an obvious nature or the testees are of sufficient attainment, or they may have to be fuller. In any case they should usually include an illustrative solution of a test of the type in question. To ensure that the testees are thoroughly familiar with the nature of the test procedure, it is often advisable to allow them to practise the solution of a few tests of each of the

---

[1] Taken from Spearman's *Measure of " Intelligence "*.

several types before they embark upon the tests by which we are going to gauge their ability. The differences between individuals in the need they have for instructions were clearly brought out in an experiment performed by the writer on school children. Each child in a class of ten-year-olds was given a pamphlet containing a pictorial " intelligence test," known as the " Otis Primary Test ". In this pamphlet are some half dozen different types of test, all depending upon the interpretation of pictures, a page of the pamphlet being devoted to each type of test. Thus, on one page is a series of pictures of objects which are incomplete in some way, such as a wheel with a spoke missing, a pistol with a trigger missing, and so on. On another page are several series of pictures, each series " telling a story ", the pictures not, however, being in the order required by the story. At the top of the page, for instance, are three pictures : the first, on the left of the page, depicts a nest with eggs in it ; to the right of this is a picture of a bird making a nest, whilst to the right of that is a picture of a nest containing little birds. The child is required to number these pictures in their order, according to the story told by the three taken together, putting 1 in the middle picture, 2 in the picture on the left, and 3 in the remaining picture. In previous experiments with this test it had been clear to me that many children realized the task they were to perform long before I had finished reading to them the very prolix Instructions provided with the test. In this experiment I went to the other extreme, giving no instructions beyond these : " On each page do what you think you are supposed to do." None of these children had ever seen these tests before, but several of them, especially those who subsequently proved themselves, in other tests, to be able children, answered many of the tests correctly.

Experiments with more advanced tests and older testees have since produced similar results. Indeed the power to read into a test, such as the story-pictures of the Otis test, a problem which has not been stated by the tester is a significant mental quality of the testee ; but it is not the quality the test is designed to indicate, and we must not, therefore, by neglecting or curtailing instructions, allow individual differences in respect of that quality to influence the test results.

5. *The Background of a Test*

Stated crudely, the method of the mental tester is to place a number of individuals in the " same situation " and then compare their reactions. But it is not merely the *objective* situation, defined by the nature of the test materials and the examiner's procedure, that must be the " same " for all the testees. What we must ensure is that the situation *as apprehended by the testees* is the same for them all. The main function of Instructions is, as we have seen, to secure this subjective similarity of test situation as between one testee and another.

Now, the subjective test situation, the testee's understanding of our tests before he solves them, is partly determined by the nature of the testee himself. His past experience and his innate qualities determine the meaning our tests have for him. According to these qualities, a given response on the part of the testee may indicate one thing or another ; according to these qualities a given test may succeed or fail in giving the indication we want it to give. Our test instructions must be given in language the testees can clearly understand ; but that is not all.[1] We must select the tests themselves so that

[1] The need for adjusting, to the ability and attainment of the person questioned, the wording of a question is, of course, familiar to teachers. See Chapter VII.

the quality we wish them to indicate [1] is the essential determinant of the responses in all the testees. Thus a geometrical theorem would be an unsatisfactory test of power of geometrical reasoning if the testees were already acquainted with the proof of the theorem. An " intelligence test " which assumes a certain background of experience in the testees (which all tests must do) fails as an indicator of " intelligence " in children who have not had that experience. If the Binet-Simon tests assume that a child has grown up in Europe or in America, and that the child has certain knowledge that is normally acquired in school and not outside school (both these statements about those tests are true), then they will not serve to indicate intelligence in a Bantu, nor will they be applicable to a European child who, for some reason, has not attended school.[2]

When we are testing *present effective ability* of any kind, we need, in designing our tests, concern ourselves only with securing that the elements of the ability are as well as possible sampled by our tests. Thus a test of power of addition of numbers should introduce all the combinations, all the cases of " carrying ", that may occur in *any* addition sum. The test we design to indicate power of writing shorthand should introduce a collection of outlines that is fairly representative of those that a person should be able without hesitation to write. If the specimen, of addition or shorthand, that the testee is required to produce, is a fair sample of the additions or shorthand passages that occur in practice, then our

---

[1] It will be convenient to refer to this as the " intended argument " of the test, or, where confusion will not arise, as simply the test's " argument ".

[2] See the account of mental testing of canal-boat children, whose attendance at school is irregular, in *Mental and Scholastic Tests among Retarded Children*, by Hugh Gordon. Board of Education (British) Educational Pamphlets, No. 44 (1923).

tests are adequate.   In interpreting the results of such tests we need know nothing about the testees except that they have in fact displayed such and such degrees of skill.   We need not know how much practice each testee has had, or how long each has been learning the skill ; we need not know whether the testee has or has not reached the limit of his proficiency ; we need not know upon what factors skill in addition or shorthand depends (except in so far as that is necessary for the proper *designing* of the tests).   For, the argument of our test is present effective ability, and *that* is indicated by the test products taken, so to speak, at their face value.

Almost always, however, we wish to use our test results as the basis of inference as to qualities of the testee which are not directly shown by those results.   We may wish to make *practical* inferences, such as that this test of the power to write this particular passage in shorthand indicates the testee's power to write *any other* passage in shorthand, or that this test of " intelligence " indicates the testee's power of intelligent thinking in *any* kind of situation.   Or, we may wish to make what might be called *theoretical* inferences, in the sense that those inferences are of interest chiefly for the contribution they make to psychological theory.   We might, for instance, wish to ascertain to what extent skill in shorthand, or the ease of learning shorthand, depends upon " intelligence ".   As a rule, when we wish to base an inference upon test results it is always necessary to interpret those results *in terms of other facts that we know about the testees.*

It is desired, we will suppose, to ascertain upon what factors skill in shorthand depends.   One interpretation of this problem would lead to an answer that was virtually an analysis of the principles of some particular form of shorthand.   Thus, in Pitman's system, the stenographer must know the shorthand alphabet, and he must know also the principles by which that alphabet is supplemented, such as the indication of the vowels by the position in which an outline is drawn—below, on or above the writing line. But a *psychological* analysis of shorthand skill reduces that skill if possible to such and such *general* mental factors—*e.g.*, perhaps kinæsthetic or visual memory, power of associating symbols and sounds, perseveration (or weakness of perseveration), power to perceive relations or certain kinds of relations, etc.—factors that are not peculiar to shorthand skill. How can we arrive at, and how verify, such an analysis? We can arrive at it partly by introspective study and partly by comparing the skill of individuals in shorthand with the degrees in which they possess the qualities upon which that skill is supposed to depend. *If* there is a general power of kinæsthetic memory, in the sense that any individual who shows that power in high degree in one kind of situation can show it in high degree in any other situation in which response depends upon such memory,[1] then we can compare an individual's skill in shorthand with his power of kinæsthetic memory as indicated by appropriate tests. And so for each of the other qualities upon which we suppose shorthand skill to be dependent. We thus interpret the individual's performance in our shorthand tests in terms of our knowledge of the degrees in which he possesses each of those other qualities.

Again, if it is ascertainable that the performance of an individual in " intelligence tests " depends partly upon

[1] In this (quantitative) statement the use of the term " such memory " begs the question of the occurrence of kinæsthetic memory in various situations. In order that there shall be any meaning in the phrase " general kinæsthetic memory," it is also necessary, of course, that there shall be a qualitative sameness between different occurrences of kinæsthetic experiences which justifies us in placing all those experiences in a single class.

innate factors and partly upon the environment in which he has grown up, we can interpret his performance in such tests only in the light of what we know about his upbringing.

6. *Width of Inference*

The practical value of any test depends chiefly upon the width of the inference we can base upon performance in the test. Such tests as those in shorthand to which we have just referred will serve, if they properly sample all the actions possible in shorthand, to indicate the individual's power to write in shorthand any word whatever. And it *is* possible to devise representative tests of shorthand skill. Most people would consider it rash, however, to draw any such general conclusions from a man's performance in shorthand as that he is likely to be quick witted, or that he is likely to be as rapid a calculator as he is a stenographer. Yet inferences of such width are quite commonly made on the basis of performance in arithmetic. The boy who is " quick at figures " is often regarded by the plain man as possessed of a general power of quick thinking, as clever in a general way. Those who believe, as Robert Recorde [1] did, that algebra is a " whetstone of wit ", may well conclude that success in an algebra test indicates in all likelihood the possession of all-round mental efficiency, or at any rate an efficiency that extends far beyond the power to solve algebraic problems.

We do not believe that the boy who excels in arithmetic necessarily excels in all other subjects, nor do we believe that the study of algebra necessarily trains our thinking power in a perfectly general way. But, on the other

---

[1] Author of a textbook of algebra, *The Whetstone of Wit*, first published in 1557.

hand, it would be hard to justify the inclusion of such a subject as algebra in the school curriculum if its study did indeed produce no effects other than the power to solve algebraic problems.   We must believe that the study of algebra in some way improves the individual's power to deal with situations differing greatly from those of algebra, if we are to retain the subject as an element of general education.   This is not the place to consider the validity of this assumption.   I wish here only to point out that, if a subject like algebra may in fact be used as an instrument for training the individual to think in non-algebraic situations, it must follow that a test in algebraic skill may indicate to some extent the testee's power outside the field of algebra.

Any test, whether it be a mental test in the usual sense of that term or an ordinary examination, must necessarily deal with a limited range of material, and can at best only require the testee to give us a fair specimen of his knowledge or his power.   The cardinal problem in mental testing is that of sampling : how, with the limitation of time and testing material to which we are perforce subject, can we best sample an individual's mental qualities ? No problem with which the mental tester is concerned is of greater importance than this, and there is none of greater complexity.   Of the importance of the problem we need give no illustration.   Its complexity is especially evident when we consider tests that purport to indicate mental qualities of considerable width.   Without pre-judice as to the meaning, or lack of meaning, of the term " intelligence ", let us see what form the problem of sampling takes in what are called " intelligence tests ".

These tests are supposed to indicate, and their whole value depends upon their power to indicate, a mental quality that enters into, or in part determines, the individual's reactions to very many situations. It is obviously quite impossible to devise a test that shall confront the testee with a representative sample of all the situations with respect to which " intelligence tests " are supposed to have a " wider indication ". " Intelligence " is supposed to enter in some degree into virtually all, if not absolutely all, cognitive reactions ; but we cannot sample all the situations to which an individual might react. Indeed a cursory survey of any intelligence test will show how very unlike problems that the individual meets in everyday life are most of the items of the test, and this fact has often been forcibly cited as evidence of their inadequacy. Now the maker of an intelligence test certainly does not attempt to sample all the objective situations with which life may confront an individual. All that he can do is to try to sample *the factors upon which reactions to all kinds of situations depend*. He has, therefore, to make the assumption that there *are* factors common to the determining causes of reaction to different kinds of situation. And this is a considerable assumption. It is an assumption that we readily make before we have given much thought to psychology : in all kinds of situations, we say, a man may have to reason, to exercise imagination, to depend upon memory, to force himself to attend to the matter in hand. Cannot our tests sample these several faculties ? But the abstraction of a general mental power, such as Reasoning or Memory, from the various particular mental processes in which we regard it as operative, is a procedure of which, as we cultivate a closer acquaintance with psychology, we become chary.[1]

---

[1] We touch here, and can do no more than touch, upon a very profound problem. In any particular instance of a reasoning process (to take the case of Reasoning) there are certain objects about which we are reasoning, and the process consists essentially in perceiving certain relations between these objects. As part of the reasoning we may, for

On the other hand, as we have seen, psychology is obliged to abstract common elements from various experiences and reactions.   The validity of a test of " general intelligence " which proceeds by attempting to sample these common elements, will depend upon the validity of the analysis leading to those elements.   To ascertain the validity of an intelligence test is thus a difficult task indeed.   And, in anticipation of the next chapter, a further difficulty may be mentioned here.   Let us suppose it possible to devise a test which fairly samples the essential factors of all kinds of thinking.   It is still true that the test cannot indicate all these factors ; it can only indicate the total effect of their conjoint action, and it may not do that.

Though the psychological basis of the wider inference we draw from the results of tests has its roots running very deep, the *fact* of " wider indication " is patent to us all.   Though we have already touched on this topic in the first chapter, the matter is of such significance in the theory of mental testing that a further illustration will not be out of place here.

In Trafalgar Square I ask a policeman to direct me to Leadenhall Street.   From his answer I may learn not only the whereabouts of Leadenhall Street, but also several things about the policeman himself.   He can

example, perceive a relation of similarity (from some standpoint) between A and B.   This process of educing a relation has, as experience, a certain special quality dependent upon the special natures of A and B ; when we describe it abstractly as a process of educing a relation of similarity we ignore that special quality.   Another experience of perceiving similarity, between, say, C and D, will have *its* special quality ; the natures of C and D enter into our thinking of this relation, but those natures do not enter into our general conception of a relation of similarity.   We ought not, then, without further evidence, to assume that power to perceive the similarity between A and B implies power to perceive that between C and D.   See Spearman : *The Abilities of Man*, pp. 38, 39 (1927).

express himself about this particular matter with a measure of clarity ; he can interpret my question, Where is Leadenhall Street ? as calling not for the latitude and longitude of the place, but for a description of its position relative to my present position ; and, if he can understand that one question, he can probably understand many others ; and if he can give clear instructions in answer to that question he could probably give equally clear instructions if he were asked to direct me to any other place with whose position he was familiar. But how far can we safely go in our inferences about the policeman ? Can we, since he can clearly picture the arrangement of streets between Trafalgar Square and Leadenhall Street, infer that he could, if given an hour to examine the street, give us an accurate description of its appearance— the kind of buildings, the nature of the road surface, and so on ?   We cannot make that inference, for the power to remember the schema of a city's streets is more specific than that of remembering all the many details that should enter into a description of the appearance of a single street.   Can we, since the London streets form a geometrical pattern, infer that the policeman could probably excel in the invention of artistic geometrical designs ? Clearly that would be too wide an inference, for, although the kind of imagery employed in recalling the arrangement of a city's streets would be of service in inventing designs, such invention also depends upon many other factors.

How can we ascertain the width of legitimate inference ? There are two broadly distinguishable ways, neither of which is adequate by itself.   Let us suppose that we wish to know whether, from the responses to a series of topographical questions, such as the one we put to our policeman, we can infer a power of visual imagery.   We can, on the one hand, devise a number of questions, the answering of which appears to depend primarily upon visual imaging, and find out empirically what degree of correlation [1] there is between the results of such tests and those of our topographical test. If there is a high degree of correlation, and if we can justify our belief that the tests of visual imagery do adequately test that power,[2] then success in the topographical test will indicate, with a certain probability, the possession of some power of visual imaging. Or, on the other hand, given an ability, such as the ability to carry in mind the schema of the streets of a city, we can attempt to discover by introspection what factors enter into this ability, and to compare these with the factors entering into our visual imagery tests. There are various reasons why this kind of introspective comparison is only crude, and why it is always liable to error. It is liable to error chiefly because the act of answering a test is never fully introspectible. But it is nevertheless a process that should always be attempted when we are endeavouring to determine the width of inference we may legitimately make upon the results of a test.

7. Classification of Tests

The process of comparing individuals by the way of mental tests has two parts. We have first to choose and define qualities with respect to which we shall effect the comparison. Then for each of these qualities we have to devise suitable tests. These two steps are not in general independent of one another. In fact, one of the aims of mental testing should be to improve our system of categories of psychological description. Thus, in order to compare the " memory ", in the sense of power of

[1] See Section 5 of Chapter III.

[2] We should first, of course, have to prove that a " general power of visual imaging "—or a " general power of visual memory "—existed.

D

recall, of individuals, we may invent various tests, the responses to all of which appear to depend chiefly upon recall. But application of the tests brings to light new facts about recall : recall, we find, may be of different kinds—an individual's power of recall may differ according to the nature of the material recalled, and he may excel in *immediate* recall but not in *delayed* recall, or *vice versa*. Tests designed to indicate *recall in general* are therefore defective ; their " intended argument " does not exist. With the results of our imperfectly designed tests in mind we effect a classification of the processes of recall, and devise, for each kind of recall, a separate set of tests. Constantly, in mental testing, we have at once to design and interpret tests in terms of our present mental categories, and to modify our categories in accordance with the findings of the tests.

In the choice of test qualities, the first of the two essential steps in testing, we are guided partly by introspection and partly by observation of the behaviour and expression of other people. Introspection reveals various kinds of mental process : sensations of the several kinds, such and such emotions, this and that kind of imaging, recall of past experience, eduction of relations, judgment, imagination, invention, insight, and so on. In such subjective analysis we are liable to many errors. Introspection, the chief aim of which is to enable us to evolve a vocabulary for psychological description, is especially liable to be influenced by our knowledge of terms already in use. Thus, the existence of the term " insight " may easily lead us to suppose that we observe an essential similarity between all experiences of insight ; and the supposition that all insightful experiences have a qualitative sameness may be correct. The degree, however, to which capacity for insight is dependent upon the material about which the thinking is concerned can only be ascertained by experiment, experiment in which mental tests will play a part. Again we find it difficult to avoid the assumption that a certain similarity between the effects of two mental processes necessarily implies an element common to the causes of those processes. Thus, the inventive processes of a poet result in a new arrangement of words, and the inventive processes of an engineer produce a new arrangement of materials. On the basis of this logical similarity between the two instances of invention, we readily assume that there is a " power of invention " which can be applied alike to words or material objects, and that the dissimilarity between the inventive thinking of the poet and that of the engineer arises solely from the fact that the first is dealing with words and the second with material objects. But this is a mode of abstraction of which we have, in an earlier paragraph, seen cause to be suspicious.

The *rôle* of mental analysis in the classifying and designing of tests will be further discussed in the next chapter. It is a large problem, upon which we can throw but a feeble candle-light. We may content ourselves here with a few elementary considerations of the possible modes of classifying tests.

Tests may be classified on one or other of several plans. In the first place we may let the subject-matter of the test be the basis of classification. This is what we generally do in " ordinary examinations " : we have tests in French, or in French grammar, or the history of French literature, in translation, and so on ; we have mathematical examinations, which again may be subdivided according to the conventional branches of mathematics ; we have tests in general science, or in any special science or section of a science. The sub-tests of which intelligence tests are composed often bear names that refer rather to their subject-matter than to the kind of mental process by which they are solved.   Thus a group test may include sub-tests entitled " Arithmetic ", " Proverbs " (in which the testee has to interpret a number of proverbs), " Synonyms " (in which from four or five words a word has to be chosen which is synonymous with a given word), " Geometric Figures " (a test containing various questions whose solution involves an analysis of a given diagram), and so on.   Although each of these sub-tests probably involves the use of mental processes peculiar to itself, the grouping of tests under such headings is primarily a matter of practical convenience ; such a grouping is not a psychological grouping ; each sub-test has value as a part of the whole test rather than because it has, taken by itself, any clear indication.

The Analogies Test, to which we have frequently referred, illustrates two kinds of classification of tests. Such a test may be regarded as defined by the form of its subject-matter : an Analogies Test is a test of the form

Kennel is to *Dog* as *House* is to . . . ?

We can then at once tell whether a given test is an Analogies Test without inquiring into the mental processes involved in its solution.   On the other hand, we may resolve the solution of such a test into two well-defined mental processes—the eduction of a relation and the eduction of a correlate.   The test may then be classified *psychologically* as a test of those mental processes.   Tests, then, may be classified according to the mental processes they evoke : eduction of relations and correlates, discrimination of musical pitch, immediate recall of visual material, geometrical reasoning, attention, judgment, and so on through the whole range of mental processes to which, rightly or wrongly, we give special names.

Finally, tests may be classified, not according to the mental processes they involve, but according to the enduring characteristics of individuals indicated : perseveration, " intelligence ", emotionality, various abilities and tendencies, capacities and attainments.

8. *Quantitative Aspects of Tests*

A mental test is a situation devised with a view to studying, under simplified conditions, the ways of thinking and otherwise reacting of individuals. As a rule we observe the *final response* (generally in the form of a written or spoken symbol) to our tests, but it is sometimes possible to observe the *process of solution*, as it was in the case of the wire puzzle, and as it is to some extent in ordinary examinations where a candidate, writing his essay or solving his problem, does some " thinking on paper ". The same final answer may often have been reached in different ways by different individuals, but we can minimize the risk of this kind of ambiguity by a suitable choice of tests, suitable test instructions, and a standardized procedure of examination. Suppose that we can devise a test of which it is possible to say, " In all likelihood any testee making the correct response to this test will think in such and such a way ". Then if several tests of this kind, which all evoke the same form of thinking, are applied to a group of individuals, what sort of individual differences will the test set as a whole indicate ? We shall notice differences in the *number* of tests individuals can answer correctly in a given time, and differences in the *difficulty* of the tests within reach of different individuals. That is to say, we shall notice *quantitative* differences between the individuals in their abilities to solve the tests. The few sidelights on mental testing to be found in the present chapter will have sufficed to show the inadequacy of the notion that mental tests are concerned *solely* with quantitative descriptions of mental qualities, a notion commonly held by laymen and perhaps too highly respected by some psychologists.   The essential characteristic of a mental test is not that it affords a measurement, a numerical description, but that, as we have reiterated, it is a situation *carefully selected or designed* with a view to eliciting responses as free as possible from ambiguity in their psychological indication. Nevertheless, the study of mental tests has from the first been closely associated with the introduction of quantitative ideas into psychology, so that " mental testing " and what has been called " mental measurement " are by many people regarded as synonymous terms.   Of such interest and significance is the concept of *measurement* in psychology that it will be discussed at some length in the next chapter.

CHAPTER III

MEASUREMENT IN PSYCHOLOGY

1. *The Approach to Measurement*

IT is not surprising that people should form strong opinions on such a question as the measurability of human qualities. On the one side, there are people in whom is a strong Pythagorean desire to give the study of human nature the definiteness of number. These people have great hopes that it may be possible to put psychology as surely as physics on a scientific basis, and they believe that science begins with measurement. On the other side are the people who assert that " human nature is too subtle and complex to be measured with a foot-rule ", that the definiteness of numerical statements stands in marked contrast to the vagueness of our knowledge of human nature. To such people the attitude of the man who attempts to state in numerical terms the degree of genius of Linnæus seems as sacrilegious as that of the man who botanizes on his own mother's grave.

There is food in plenty for prejudice both for and against mental measurement. The ardent advocate of mental measurement can point to its many undoubted successes in education, industry, and pure psychology. His opponent, however, who wishes to disprove the possibility of such measurement, has been generously supplied by " psychologists " with unwarranted deductions from the results of mental testing, so that if the sceptic chooses his victims carefully he can maul them as much as he wishes.

The hope of the extremist in quantitative psychology is to obtain measurements of the differences between individuals in respect of all the various kinds of mental qualities : intelligence, emotionality, originality, ascendance over or submission to other people, knowledge, abilities of all types, amorousness, power of appreciating or of composing music, sensory acuity, and so on. It is true that there must be a qualitative analysis of mind before we can know what are the qualities with respect to which we can compare people. But even here the mathematical psychologist can make out a plausible case for the possibility of effecting such analysis by statistical methods.

Measurement consists in the assignment, under certain conditions, of numbers to the qualities of things. Measured qualities must therefore have a definite *order*, the order of the numbers assigned to them.   They must also have other properties, but we will consider the property of order first.

In our description of mental qualities we have continually to use comparative terms. The phrases of everyday psychology afford abundant illustrations of this. " I am much happier than I was yesterday "; " The pain is less acute than it was " ; " Jones is the man of more force of character, but Smith has the greater sense of humour " ; " The Astronomer Royal requires more intelligence than an unskilled labourer " ; " The wisdom of Socrates was greater than that of Xantippe "; " A sadder and a wiser man " ; and so *ad infinitum*. Here we have several instances of qualities that can in a sense be judged greater or less than others of like kind. And where we have qualities such that any one is greater or less than every other of the same kind, those qualities must have a serial order. We can imagine a pain, for example, to grow from a barely perceptible sensation to acute agony, passing through all the intermediate stages in their definite serial order. Again, we can certainly say of two men that one has more knowledge or greater ability of a given kind than the other. In fact, we often arrange a number of examination candidates in what is supposed to be the order of their amounts of knowledge or ability. Knowledge, ability, or sensations, whether or not they are measurable in the strict sense of the word, have at least this much resemblance to qualities, such as weights, that are admittedly measurable : namely, that they have a definite order, or that they enable us to arrange men in a definite order, just as a number of objects may be arranged in the order of their weights.

Belief in the possibility of measuring mental qualities— sensations, tendencies, capacities—is encouraged by the fact that the *behaviour and expression* by which mental qualities are indicated most certainly *have* quantitative aspects. Thus, in behaviour we have speed and accuracy of movement ; we have, for instance, the speed and accuracy with which a man can use a typewriter. A man's typewriting speed and accuracy can be expressed in numbers, and the same is true of very many human actions. Whether or not it is possible to measure the intensity of a man's sensation, there is often no difficulty in the measurement of his power to discriminate between the intensities of sensory stimuli. We may ascertain the number of vibrations per second by which two musical notes (at any given part of the scale) must differ in order that a person shall be able to recognize the notes as of different pitches ; we find that power of pitch discrimination so measured varies from person to person, but is practically constant in any one person. At the note of Middle C, for example, many people can observe the difference between notes whose vibrations differ by four, whilst some can detect a difference of less than one vibration. We may express in physical units an individual's power to discriminate between lights or pressures of nearly equal intensities. Again, we can compare the speeds with which individuals can correctly calculate, or the accuracies with which they can shoot. And whatever may be the psychological significance of the numbers obtained, we can compare the numbers of items in an " intelligence test " correctly answered by different testees.

The existence of continuously graded qualities, such as sensations, and the possibility of expressing numerically certain aspects of human action, such as quantity of work done, both suggest that measurement in some sense may be possible in psychology. With the essential nature of measurement we have no call to deal in this book. Our concern will be, not so much with the question, Are " mental measurements " really measurements ? as with the question, How may the numbers obtained in mental testing to be interpreted ? In our attempt to answer the latter question, however, we shall incidentally, it is hoped, throw some light on the former. By the term " mental measurements " we shall often mean no more than " numbers obtained in mental testing." Ever since psychologists first attempted to introduce numerical statements into their science, the term " mental measurement " has been acquiring a wider and wider meaning, and there is some danger that this fact should be forgotten ; there is some danger that, for example, the unwary should suppose that " intelligence " can be " measured " in the sense that weight or length can be measured. With ebullient energy psychologists have eagerly frequented schools and clinics, universities and business houses, " measuring " this mental quality and that, with a confidence that would be admirable were it not the confidence that comes of wearing blinkers. And thus "mental measurement" has so extended its scope (including now even such qualities as "moral sense" or "sense of beauty") that the humble parents of quantitative psychology would hardly recognize the fat, prosperous individual into whom their child has grown ; nor, perhaps, would they be proud of him.

2. *Psychophysics*

The brilliant success with which measurement had been applied to the establishment of physical laws was the main cause of the eagerness with which psychologists in the middle and later nineteenth century attempted to measure mental qualities. And, drawing their inspiration from physics, they started their inquiries as near to physics as possible. They set themselves to measure sensation. It was their hope that they might lay the foundations of all psychology in the study of sensation, and that they might discover quantitative laws descriptive of sensations and other mental phenomena.

With the methods and results of these psychophysicists, as they were appropriately called, we have no space and no call to deal. They did not succeed in solving the problem they set out to solve. But their failure was fruitful and left a valuable legacy of clearly defined problems ; it made evident the need for an inquiry into the nature of measurement in general, and created the opportunity for an enlargement of our conception of measurement. Thus it became clear from their researches that sensation intensity, if indeed it is a magnitude at all, differs in a fundamental respect from such magnitudes as length, which can be expressed as containing so many units. For, the intensity of a sensation is not, as experience, divisible into units. We may be aware that the light given by a hundred candles is of the same intensity as that given by one electric bulb, but we cannot *experience* the brighter light as composed of a hundred duller lights, in the way that we can experience the length of a foot as composed of twelve inches. It is idle to say that the hundred duller lights are present in the one brighter light, although we cannot experience the brighter light as composed of them, for it is *experience* that we are trying to measure. In the sense, then, of consisting of so many units sensation is not measurable.

But can we so enlarge the concept of " measurement " that " intensive magnitudes ", such as sensation, may be regarded as measurable ? Consider first a collection of magnitudes that are measurable in the ordinary sense— such as a number of lengths. These may, in the first place, be arranged in order of magnitude. So also can a number of sensations of light be arranged in the order of their intensities. But in addition to the relations of greater and less which enable us to arrange our lengths into their order of magnitude, there are other relations between the lengths. We can say that each length contains so many units, and that two lengths differ in magnitude by the difference in the numbers of the units they contain. Thus, taking a length of three feet and a length of five feet, the larger length may be regarded as containing two parts, of which one is the smaller length of three feet and the other is the difference of two feet. Now, there clearly cannot be such relations of difference between two intensities of sensation, for the larger of the two cannot be conceived as divisible into parts. Nevertheless, we are aware of a relation between any two sensation intensities, which, though it is not the difference between the two intensities, is definitely fixed by their magnitudes. It is a relation of difference between the two intensities, but it is not the difference between them in the sense of an intensity which added to the smaller produces the larger. Call it the " distance " between the intensities. This " distance " is itself a kind of magnitude, for we can say that one " distance " is larger or smaller than another. If we have three sensation intensities (of light-sensation, we will suppose), A, B, and C, we can say that the distance between A and B is greater than, equal to, or less than the distance between B and C. This gives us the clue to the problem of enlarging the concept of measurement. For, if the distance AB is equal to the distance BC, we can *agree to call* the distance AC twice the distance AB. If, again, the distance CD, between C and a fourth intensity, D, of the same kind, is equal to AB and BC, we can agree to say that the distance AD is three times the distance AB. This convention provides us with a means of measuring *distances*, and we may further agree that the intensities themselves, A, B, C, etc., shall be regarded as measured by their distances, in terms of the unit AB, from the intensity A.[1]

The psychophysicists did not get so far as this. Indeed they made palpable errors, owing to their neglect of the fact that intensities are indivisible and cannot therefore be added to or subtracted from one another after the manner of lengths or weights. But their labours directed attention to the special problems involved in the "measurement " of intensities, and have in several ways influenced the development of mental testing.

3. *Psychostatistics*

We turn now to a type of " measurement " which differs considerably from that of psychophysics. Most of

---

[1] See Bertrand Russell: *Principles of Mathematics* (1903).

the " mental measurements " of the present day are essentially nothing more than *counts of the test items correctly answered by an individual.* Of this type are the measurements immediately yielded by all " intelligence tests ". The usual procedure is to assign a score of unity to each test item (each Analogy, each arithmetical problem, each sentence to be completed or each word to be fitted into a sentence, and so on). The total score is the number of items correctly answered. This " raw score " is then generally manipulated in some way—*e.g.*, it may be divided by the average score for individuals of the same age as the testee—and the number so obtained is the " measurement " furnished by that test. This kind of measurement, and others that may be grouped with it in the class of " statistical measurements ", are the kinds we shall chiefly have in mind in the remainder of this chapter.

A full discussion of the nature of statistical measurement would involve the introduction of mathematics which, whilst it would simplify my task, would not perhaps simplify my reader's. We will content ourselves with exploring some of the forms such measurements may take, and some of the more obvious principles governing their interpretation.

The simplest case of such measurement is that already mentioned : the count of correct test responses. Any interpretation of such a score must rest upon the assumption that all the separate items, since each of them receives the same score (viz., unity), are in some way (*e.g.*, in " difficulty ") equivalent to one another. If this kind of score is to be free from ambiguity it must moreover be possible to divide all answers to any given test item into two classes—that of correct, and that of incorrect, answers. It must not be possible for various answers to an item to have different *degrees of correctness*. In this kind of measurement the only indication of differences between testees lies in differences in their *total* score. The score may indicate either the number of items the testee can correctly answer in a given time, or the number he is capable of answering when there is no time limit.

When a test item, such as the Ball and Field test to which we have already alluded, may evoke answers of various degrees of goodness, we may score it in either of two ways. We first arrange all the possible answers in order of their goodness. We may then draw a line, somewhere in this series of answers, dividing the " correct " from the " incorrect " answers ; or, we may divide the answers into several classes, and assign 1, 2, 3, . . . marks to an answer according to the class into which it falls. If the latter procedure is adopted, the mark assigned to an answer indicates the merit of that answer *as a whole*. Thus, if an answer to the Ball and Field test is deemed to have four " units " of merit, we must not ask what part or aspect of the answer earns each of these units.

An allied type of statistical measurement consists in the comparison of the degree of merit of a test product with the merits of the products of a large number of individuals. Thus it may be possible to arrange a large number of essays in an order of merit about which a considerable consensus of opinion may be obtained. A further essay may now be compared with this series and scored according to the position it appears to occupy in the series. The score then represents the merit of the essay *as a whole ;* it is not the sum of a number of part scores, each of which is assignable to some part or some aspect of the essay. Such a " measurement ", of course, depends greatly upon the examiner's power of judgment, as well as upon the candidate's power of essay writing. Since the merit of the essay is here regarded as an indivisible whole, its indication by numbers is comparable with the " measurement " of a sensation intensity.

There are other modes of statistical measurement, but no purpose would be served by enumerating them. In all such measurement, test products (the answers to an " intelligence test ", or any other psychological test, or to a test in mathematics or English or any other subject) are numerically assessed according to some scheme, *and the numbers so obtained are then regarded as measuring some mental quality of the testee.* The score assigned to a product will *usually* be the sum of a number of part scores (of the scores, namely, for separate test items or examination questions or parts of examination questions), but the score, considered as a whole, is supposed to indicate the value of some single mental quality. This brings us to a fundamental principle which governs every kind of measurement.

4. *The Principle of the Single Variable*

However numerous may be the causes that combine to produce a test response, or however many aspects of a test product we may review in forming a general estimate of its value, we must not overlook the fact that the test score, being a single number, can only represent a single fact. The temperature of a sick man may be the joint product of many causes, but it is itself a single thing ; there is no sense in which it can be regarded as a " joint measure " of the several causes. The capacity of a cistern depends upon three things, the length, the breadth, and the depth of the cistern. But the capacity is a single quantity which is not a length, nor yet three lengths.

That quantity could, in fact, be ascertained by means of a gallon measure in a manner that involved no direct reference to length at all. Again, the sum of the length and breadth of an oblong does not " jointly measure " the length and breadth. It measures the semi-perimeter, a single variable with a clear meaning of its own, quite independent of the meanings of length and breadth. The product of the length and the breadth measures another single variable, the area. On the other hand, if we add the numbers specifying perimeter and area respectively, we obtain a number that cannot be regarded as measuring any definite property of the oblong.

The truth that a single number can represent only a single fact, which seems so trite when we are talking about cisterns and oblongs, is sometimes forgotten when people talk about minds. When, for instance, it is desired to measure a man's proficiency in some complex activity, such as engineering, what is generally done is to set him a number of diverse tests—in the theory of machines, the principles of mechanics and practical mathematics, perhaps some science, perhaps some surveying, and other forms of activity incidental to the engineer's profession. The total of marks from all these tests is then taken as a measure of his proficiency in the engineering activity as a whole. In point of practice this procedure may be justified, but we have a flagrant example of the fallacy we are discussing when the total (or the average of the marks in the separate tests, which comes to the same thing) is said to represent the man's skill in all the activities tested. Again, we award scholarships on the total of marks obtained in a number of different subjects, regarding this total as measuring the candidate's merit " on the whole ". Now, there may be a meaning in the phrase " merit on the whole ", if there is a common

E

factor which is part cause of all the diverse abilities whose measures are totalled, for the total mark may then, on certain assumptions, be regarded as measuring that common factor. But if, on the contrary, the various abilities are really quite independent of one another, then there is no meaning in the phrase " merit on the whole ", and the total marks, or the average mark, must be regarded as being without definite psychological significance.

If a person takes a test involving several different kinds of task, his total score does not " jointly measure " the abilities involved in working those tasks. There appear to be two things that such a total might measure. If the whole series of tasks *is* in some sense a whole, and not, like most intelligence tests, a congeries of disparate items, then there may be said to be an ability associated with the test as a whole, and the total measures that ability, though it gives no indication of the magnitudes of the component abilities. Thus, if we give so many marks for various processes in the making of a chair, we may, on certain assumptions, say that the total of these marks gives a measure of the power to make a chair. We may say that such and such components enter into the total chair-making ability, that they have respectively such and such importance, and we may allow them to contribute to the total mark in proportion to their importance. Here many causes lead to one total effect. On the other hand we may have, as in the case of an intelligence test, a total score obtained by the addition of the scores of many diverse component tests, there being no unitary or whole ability that the set of tests as a whole can be said to measure. There may, however, be a *common factor* running through all the component tests and, on certain assumptions, it may be possible for us to suppose that the total test score measures the magnitude of this common factor.

A single score, if it is to have any clear meaning as a psychological measurement, must represent the magnitude of some single, homogeneous variable. The score must not be a mere total of the scores for a number of disparate tests ; disparate in the sense that there is nothing in common to the mental processes by which they are solved, or to the causes of those mental processes. If Smith makes a score of 30 points, and Jones makes 50 points, in a test, the essential cause of Smith's 30 must be qualitatively the same as the essential cause of Jones's 50. This implies two things. It implies that any given test item is solved by the same mental process by all the testees who answer it ; and that all the mental processes by which the various test items are solved have a common element, or at least that there is some *common cause* which is a partial determinant of all those mental processes. Thus, we must not have one testee answering a test item chiefly by the aid of memory, and another answering the same item chiefly by reasoning ; nor must we include in the same total the score for two tests (for the sake of illustration, say an Analogies Test and an Arithmetic Test), unless there is a factor common to the causes of responses to the two tests, and unless that factor is the chief determinant of the total obtained by adding the scores of the two tests. In short, a test must *measure the same thing in all the testees*, and all component parts of the test must measure, or contribute to the measurement of, that same thing.

This last clause calls for an illustration. But though the principle we are discussing is so fundamental, it is hard to find an illustration that is free from ambiguity. An Analogies Test, considered by itself regardless of whether or not it is part of a wider " intelligence test ", may perhaps be taken as an instance of a test, each item of which measures " the same thing ". It measures the power to educe relations and correlates. But even here an assumption is made when we regard the total score for Analogies as a measurement. For, relations have many kinds and may be educed between many kinds of things. If it were found empirically that power to educe one kind of relation is generally proportional to the same individual's power to educe all other kinds of relation, if power to educe relations were, moreover, independent of the materials between which the relations were educed, then certainly the total score could be regarded as measuring that power. But if, on the other hand, it were found that different kinds of relation were educed by different powers, so that a man might excel in the eduction of one kind of relation yet be deficient in another kind, then the total score of an Analogies Test involving various types of relation would be of ambiguous psychological significance. The addition of scores of tests that had no kind of connection with one another (could such tests be devised) could only produce a quite meaningless total, comparable, for example, to the sum of a man's stature, his girth, his age and his income. By a piece of good fortune it rarely happens, and according to some inquirers it never happens, that two tests, or the causes of the responses to two tests, are wholly unrelated with one another.

5. *Correlation and Factors*

A correlation measure is a number that shows the degree to which two kinds of statistics tend to increase or decrease together. If it is said that there is a positive correlation between arithmetic and English composition, what is meant is that those testees who score high marks in arithmetic are likely to score high marks in composition also ; that if the testees were arranged in the order of their marks in arithmetic, and then rearranged themselves into the order of their marks in composition, there would be a correspondence, close if the correlation is high, between the two orders.

The study of functional relationships between physical variables (more strictly, the functional relationships to which physical correlations so closely correspond) has been the mainspring of progress in physics. In psychology we can have few, if any, laws expressible in mathematical formulæ. The variables we measure in psychology, though never functionally related, are nevertheless generally correlated. All the theories of mind that have been put forward on the basis of the results of mental testing have been devised with a view to accounting for the correlations between the scores of different tests.

Suppose that two tests (a test, for instance, in the addition of numbers and one in subtraction) show a correlation : to what shall we attribute the correlation ? The score in each test made by any individual is the joint product of many causes, or " factors," as they are usually, perhaps not very happily, called. The correlation occurs because some of these determining factors are operative both in the addition test and in the subtraction. Thus both adding and subtracting depend upon knowledge of number combinations, such as $7 + 5 = 12$, and, if they are written tests and employ numbers of more than one digit, both will involve some understanding of notation. Apart from such evident common factors there are doubtless others of a more obscure nature, including some factors of a purely physiological nature that cannot possibly be known introspectively.

Where the subject-matter of one test has obviously much in common with that of a second test, as in the case of addition and subtraction, we expect to find that the two tests are correlated. But even the most diverse tests generally show some degree of correlation. The writer applied to school children tests including such widely different operations as addition, cancelling all the A's in several lines of printed letters, completing the drawing of a symmetrical figure (given half of the figure) and other tests. There was correlation between every one of these tests and every other one. And numerous experiments have been carried out by many investigators with the same result : namely, that practically all tests, however disparate they may appear, are positively correlated with one another ; that is to say, there is indicated by test results a decided *tendency* for a man who is of more than average ability in one kind of performance to be of more than average ability in every other kind of performance. Can some explanation be offered of this universality of correlation ?

Any attempt to " explain " such a state of affairs involves two steps. The first step is mathematical. We take a group of individuals and subject them to a series of mental tests of many diverse kinds. The scores of the various tests display certain correlations. The first step is to invent a system of factors by which such correlations might be generated. Thus, if four abilities were all intercorrelated, we might invent the hypothesis that the scores A, B, C, D of the tests were due to the action of five factors P, Q, R, S, T according to the scheme :—

A is produced by (P, Q, R)
B   ,,   ,,   (Q, R, S)
C   ,,   ,,   (R, S, T)
D   ,,   ,,   (S, T, P).

This scheme would produce a correlation between each ability and each of the three other abilities. Again, we might propose the following simpler scheme,[1] in which all the correlations are due to the operation of the *same* factor :—

$$A \text{ is produced by (P, G)}$$
$$B \quad ,, \quad ,, \quad (Q, G)$$
$$C \quad ,, \quad ,, \quad (R, G)$$
$$D \quad ,, \quad ,, \quad (S, G).$$

And other schemes might be devised. This mathematical game is the first step in the interpretation of correlations. But there remains the second step, without which the first is indeed a mere " game ". Assuming that our scheme of factors is what gives rise to the observed correlations, we must then try to ascertain the *nature* of each of the factors. Thus, if the second of the two schemes given above is the hypothesis adopted, there are several questions concerning the nature of G that we might then set ourselves to solve. For example :—

(1) Is G a psychological factor such as " power of voluntary attention " or " power of educing relations ", etc. ? This kind of interpretation is subject to the danger that attends all attempts to abstract " general powers ", a difficulty to which we have already referred.[2]

(2) Is G to be regarded as a factor that exists " side by side " with the specific factors P, Q, R, S, or does it in some way combine with P, Q, R, S to produce A, B, etc. ?

---

[1] In a series of papers and books which are landmarks in the history of mental testing, Spearman has advocated a theory of this form. Though it appears to the writer that Spearman's theory is the most acceptable of those that have been put forward, this " Theory of Two Factors " is here given merely for illustration and without prejudice as to its probability or the contrary.

[2] See p. 46.

In chemical analogy, is each of the abilities a mixture of two factors or a compound of them ?

(3) Is G possibly a purely physiological quantity, dependent, for example, upon the structure of the nervous system or upon the secretions of the ductless glands ?

(4) If some abilities clearly depend upon G to a greater extent than others do, can we get any insight into the probable nature of G by a psychological examination of the abilities in which the influence of G is greatest ?

We need pursue this kind of speculation no further. The cardinal principle I wish to make clear is that any " theory of factors " is a piece of pure mathematics so long as it is not supplemented by a theory as to the nature of the factors. There is a considerable danger in psycho-statistics lest, by thinking overmuch in terms of factors that are only statistically defined, we shall get further and further away from the psychological realities that lie behind our test results ; and then we shall find that there is no health in us.

6. Definition of Test Arguments [1]

If a mental tester wants to hit his mark he must take as careful an aim as possible when designing his tests. He must, before he makes his measuring instrument, define, as well as conditions allow, the variable he intends to measure. It is true that tests must in the first place often be designed with only very rough notions as to the nature of what they are intended to measure ; [2] it is true that the trying out of tests based upon such approximate notions is one means of reaching clearer ideas which can then become the basis of design of further tests ; it

---

[1] For meaning of " Argument," see p. 41.
[2] Cp. Section 7 of Chapter II.

is true that we can often use such terms as " attention ", " reasoning ", " intelligence ", etc., in everyday life to good purpose although we are furnished with no adequate definitions of them ; but it is also true that progressive precision of definition of what is being measured by his tests is a duty that the psychologist must not shirk.

The chief purpose of the definition of a measured variable is to control the interpretation we are likely to put upon tests that go by the name used in the definition. Thus if we define a test as a test of " memory ", the implication is that the test measures an individual's power of recall, regardless of the nature of the recalled material, of the method by which the material was learnt, or of the time that has elapsed since the learning of the material. That is to say, it is implied that nature of material, method of learning, and time since learning have no effect upon the " memory " which is measured by our test. If this assumption proves erroneous, we shall have to delimit the interpretation that can be put upon the test results by saying that the measure provided by the test is that of the individual's power of remembering such and such material, learnt by a certain procedure and recalled after a given time.

The extreme difficulty of framing such delimiting definitions of what tests measure has led some investigators, who nevertheless make and use tests, virtually to neglect altogether the task of definition on the plea, which cannot be approved, that it is of no importance. That position has been maintained more especially in connection with " intelligence tests ". It is so terribly hard to find a definition of " intelligence " that would suit the tastes of everybody that some psychologists have given up the attempt, openly declaring that they were not interested in the matter. They then proceed to define " intelligence " as " what these particular tests measure ". Now, it is clear that this is illegitimate ; if " intelligence " is defined merely as what certain kinds of tests measure, then it is not psychologically defined at all. And in point of fact nobody can design tests to measure an " intelligence " that is defined in that way. The very psychologists who pretend indifference to the task of definition include some kinds of test, and reject others, in the design of their test-series. But they lazily refrain from analysing the grounds of their selection.

Tests should always when possible be defined *by the argument they are intended to measure.*[1] A test must not be called a test of intelligence *because* it contains Analogies, Opposites, Disarranged Sentences, Classification Tests, and the rest of the conventional repertoire of the mental tester.   On the contrary the inclusion of these items in the test is justifiable only on the grounds that they probably afford some indication of an " intelligence " of which we have some notion, however tentative it may be. We may suppose that " power to deal with new situations " is an adequate definition of " intelligence ", and then justify the inclusion of Analogies in our test-series because they present the testee with a situation that is likely to be new to him. Or, we may prefer to regard intelligence as " the power of abstract thinking ", and justify our test items because each of them calls for some feat of abstraction. Suppose it is now discovered that there is no general unitary " power to deal with new situations " ; then (quite apart from the fact that " new situations " is itself a term needing rigorous definition) the definition of our test argument is defective. We shall then be wrong in supposing that an individual's score in the test measures

---

[1] Is it not better, at any rate for elementary purposes, to say that " A ruler is an instrument for measuring length ", than to say " Length is that which is measured by a ruler " ?

his power to deal with *all kinds* of "new situations". Similarly if a man's power of abstract thinking in one kind of situation or with one kind of material is not correlated with his power of abstract thinking in all other situations and with all other kinds of material, a test defined as a test of "power of abstract thinking" is ambiguously defined. It purports to have a wider indication than in fact it has.[1] It may be said to suffer from an "*error of definition*".

7. *Errors in Testing*

The main theme of any theory of measurement is an account of the nature of errors. When a physicist is telling you how to use an instrument, his description generally consists largely in pointing out the many ways in which you may misuse it. I remember, when first making during the War a close study of the practical use of the sextant, being very familiar with the many ways in which it could get out of order before I had any clear idea of how it was to be used. Measurement is still more of a comedy—or tragedy—of errors in psychology than in other sciences.

When a physicist makes a measurement he takes various precautions against error. The psychologist measuring, for example, intelligence or memory, would fain take precautions as the physicist does. But he is handicapped by considerations with which the physicist is never troubled. For, it may seem a comparatively simple matter (it is not always so simple as it seems) for the physicist to know whether a given cause affecting his measurements is an irrelevant, disturbing factor, or is part and parcel of the thing he is trying to measure.[2] But it

[1] Cp. Ch. I, Section 7, and Ch. II, Section 6.
[2] See *Measurement and Calculation*, by Norman R. Campbell (1928).

is far more difficult for the psychologist to know what causes are influencing his measurements, and far more difficult to discriminate between causes that are intrinsic to the measurement he wishes to make and causes that are extrinsic, " interference factors ".

In the task of discriminating between intrinsic and extrinsic factors in mental measurement common sense will carry us a long way. If, for example, we wish to measure memory for patterns which are shown to the testee for a brief interval, it will clearly be necessary to make sure that none of the testees suffer from uncorrected defects of vision. We must further ensure, if possible, that all the testees are doing their best, and are not allowing their attention to wander during the exposure of the patterns ; for, we want to measure the maximum power of which the testee is capable (anything less than that is an indefinite quantity, since he may give very many degrees of attention less than his maximum to the matter, with as many degrees of success in remembering the patterns). If there is any form of distraction, either peculiar to an individual (such as illness or nervousness) or common to all the testees (such as a noise), the test will be defective—*unless*, in the case of the noise, the argument of the test is " power of visual memorizing with an auditory distraction ". Again, if there is reason to suppose that visual memory can be trained, our test will suffer from an " error of definition " unless we qualify the definition of the argument : we might describe the test as a measure of " maximum power of visual memorizing which, with training, an individual can acquire ".

But common sense cannot in detail define the width of indication it is possible to associate with a test. If a test, consisting of a number of nonsense syllables slowly spoken to the testee, then to be reproduced, is called a

" test of auditory memory ", we can only ascertain by experiment whether the test also indicates the testee's power to reproduce *other* heard material, such as melodies or spoken numbers.

Physicists recognize a distinction between " systematic errors " and " accidental errors ". An inaccurately poised balance will give rise to systematic errors, which will affect all the measurements taken. So also a measuring scale in which the " inches " were in fact 1·01 inches long would give rise to a systematic error in all measurements. But the draughts that blow the balance, or the dust that settles on the pans whilst the measurement is taking place produce accidental errors, which may affect some measurements considerably and others little if at all.

In psychological measurement similarly we may have both systematic and accidental errors. An " error of definition ", for example, is analogous to the systematic error of physics, for it affects the measurement, or the interpretation of the measurement, of *every individual tested*. But, whereas in the case of the ill-poised balance, there is no doubt that the systematic error *is* an error, the psychologist (since what he is trying to measure is never so clearly defined as mass or weight) is often not certain whether to include a given factor amongst the *essential determinants* of the test's argument or amongst the causes of *error*. Shall he, for example, regard such distractions as noises as interference factors in a test intended to measure " power of attention " ? According to one interpretation of " attention ", the very power to think in spite of distractions is part of or one aspect of " attention ". On the other hand those who can give the closest " attention " to what they have in hand, in another sense of the term " attention ", are frequently very sensitive to disturbing noises.

Of " interference factors ", in the sense of factors leading unmistakably to errors of measurement, it is easy to give any number of instances. Some of these, such as illness or nervousness, may be peculiar to individual testees, or may operate in a few testees but not in all. Some, such as errors of definition, or errors due to ambiguous instructions, may affect our measurements of all the individuals. If, during a test of power of computation, there are, in the case of some or all testees, such factors as anxiety, emotional bias against the test, or fatigue, we must reckon these as interference factors ; for they are not always present when calculations are performed, and their presence during the test will therefore prevent us from knowing how well the testees can calculate under normal conditions—which is what we generally want to know.   Sometimes, however, tests of computation are used in the measurement of fatigue, and fatigue is then no longer an interference factor.   Again, if a test is intended to be a test of *capacity*, the past experience of the testees, if it varies in amount from person to person, will act as an interference factor. We cannot compare individuals with respect to their capacity, by merely inspecting their present attainments whilst ignoring the fact that some have had every opportunity of developing their powers, and others have had none.   We cannot test the potentialities of a Milton, whose upbringing has hitherto kept him mute and inglorious, by asking him to write a *Paradise Lost*.

It is possible for a test to measure what it was intended to measure in some individuals, but to measure something else or nothing at all in others.   In such a case the test suffers from error of definition in the case of the last-named persons, but not in that of the first.   Any test, for example, suffers from error of definition if the " instructions " are not suited to the testees : for though it is supposed to measure their power to solve certain problems, the test scores are determined, not by that power, but by the power to understand the instructions, a power which may vary from individual to individual.

8. *The Validity of Tests*

The validity of a mental test — its freedom from error—is ultimately ascertainable by comparing the performance of individuals in the test with their subsequent performances (in situations similar to the test situation or not).   Or it may be approximately estimated by comparing the test results with judgments of the abilities of the individuals by competent judges.   This method of " validation " by comparing test results with " subjective judgments " of the abilities of the testees has frequently been employed in the case of " intelligence tests ".   The theory of the process seems to be somewhat as follows.   A number of " competent judges " place in order of intelligence a group of individuals, which may be called the calibration group.   An " intelligence test " is then applied, and if its scores place the individuals in the same order as the judgment-order, then the test is valid ; if the orders differ, then the test is deemed to be not valid.   Subsequently an individual, not belonging to the calibration group, scores x points in the test.   If the test is valid, then the judges, if without the test they were to judge the intelligence of that individual, would agree in giving him x points.

Now it is clear that such a mode of checking the validity of tests is at best a makeshift.   And this for several reasons.   In the first place, the judges by whose subjective judgments (of the intelligence, or other test argument, of the testees in the calibration group) the validity of the test is decided, must certainly be in some sense *competent*. But in defining a " competent judge " it seems impossible to avoid circularity : a competent judge is one who can judge " intelligence ", and a test is said to measure " intelligence " when its findings agree with those of a " competent judge " ! The principal objection to the procedure is that it in no way advances our understanding of the nature of " intelligence ". The procedure is acceptable without question only if the judges agree amongst themselves and with psychologists in general as to the nature of " intelligence ". But in proportion as that agreement is possible, so is it possible for the judges to gauge the validity of the tests *by inspecting them*, and without forming independent judgments of the mental qualities of the individuals of a calibration group. In proportion, on the other hand, as the nature of intelligence is only obscurely known, light may certainly be thrown upon the probable validity, and upon the practical value, of the tests by comparing their results with any other information about the testees—such as the so-called " subjective judgments " of their " intelligence " by a number of persons who have had opportunity of forming opinions, by the everyday methods to which reference has been made in our first chapter, of the mental qualities of the testees.

When our tests are looked upon, rather as instruments for the furtherance of our psychological knowledge than as devices for the practical, approximate discrimination of individual differences, we need to know, not merely whether the objective findings of the tests will be borne out by the subsequent performance of the testees, but also upon what hypothesis of the nature of mind the test results can be explained ; and the question of the validity of the tests is then inseparably bound up with that of the validity of our psychological hypothesis.

There are two methods, only broadly distinguishable from one another, of gauging the validity of mental tests. The first of these may be called the empirical method. It is applicable with least danger of error to tests that are frankly designed with a view more to meeting the needs of practical life than to furthering research in pure psychology. A number of tests, for example, have been devised to facilitate the selection of individuals for particular kinds of occupation ; or again for diagnosing the aptitudes of individuals in order to assist them in their choice of a vocation. They are designed in the hope that they will indicate who, amongst a number of individuals, will probably make the best tinker, tailor, soldier or sailor ; or in the hope that they will help young persons to decide whether their bent lies in the direction of the sword or the plough. If the tests prove to have high prognostic value, if, that is to say, the discriminations they effect are borne out by the subsequent careers of the testees, then they have fulfilled their aim ; in other words, they are valid. We must, of course, in order to ascertain the validity of such tests, have some means of gauging success in the vocations with respect to which they are supposed to have prognostic value. But such success is commonly not hard to measure.

" Intelligence tests " (though they generally form part of the outfit of the vocational tester) present a strong contrast to the tests we have just mentioned. The " vocation " to which intelligence tests have reference is life itself. The great width of their indication renders it extremely difficult to apply the empirical method of validation to them, and we are unable to dispense with the more fundamental method of *analysis*. The tests

F

must, introspectively and statistically, be analysed, and an attempt made to define as clearly as possible the nature of the single *psychological* variable they measure. The empirical method can only justify us in specifying an *objective* variable (such as success in a particular occupation) which is measured by a given test.

9. *Recapitulation*

In this and the previous chapter I have attempted to describe a few of the general principles underlying the use and interpretation of mental tests. With the details of tests or with the results that have been obtained by their application we have not been directly concerned. The main principles (not all mutually independent) introduced into the two chapters are as follows :—

(1) A mental test, in the broadest sense of the term, is any situation to which we observe the reactions of a number of individuals ; more particularly, a situation designed with a view to comparing individuals with respect to a given mental quality.

(2) A mental test must present the *same* problem to all the testees ; the problem must be interpreted by the testee in the sense intended by the examiner.

(3) It must be possible for an examiner to infer from a testee's success in a test, that the testee experienced certain mental processes, so that success must indicate the same kind of mental process in all the individuals who succeed.

(4) This implies that any one test item must have only one correct answer.

(5) To secure condition (2) the Instructions given to the testees before they solve the tests must be suited to the ability and attainments of the testees.

(6) The tests must be designed so that the mental quality we wish to measure is the main determinant of the testees' responses.

(7) The value of a test depends upon its power to indicate a mental quality that enters into, or in part determines, the individual's reactions to many situations, many of them often differing considerably from the test situation.

(8) Tests may be classified according to their subject-matter, according to the mental processes they evoke, or according to the enduring characteristics of the testee in virtue of which he makes his responses.

(9) The results of mental tests are generally, but not necessarily always, expressed in numerical terms. The most frequently employed kind of " mental measurement " consists essentially of a count of test items correctly answered by a testee.

(10) We can measure only one thing at a time ; one number can represent the magnitude of only one quantity. Hence a mental test has clear significance only if there is some single psychical variable whose value it may be supposed to indicate.   The test must accordingly measure the same thing in all the testees.

(11) The significance of mental test results has hitherto been arrived at chiefly by the use of correlation. The existence of correlations between various abilities is generally explained by one or other scheme of " factors " which, by combining in various ways, produce the correlated abilities. The theory of the mathematical arrangement of the factors must be supplemented by a theory of their psychological nature.

(12) When possible, tests should be defined by the argument they are intended to measure. If a test is

intended to measure a variable X, and actually it measures a different variable, Y, or measures nothing definite at all, then it suffers from an error, which it is proposed to call an " error of definition ", which affects the measurement of all the testees.

(13) A test, however, may be free from errors of definition when it is applied to one set of testees, yet fail, through error of definition, to measure the intended variable in another set. It may be necessary to employ different tests to measure a given variable, X, according to the nature of the testees. Thus, in an attempt to measure " intelligence " we shall have to use one or another kind of test, or to modify our test Instructions, according to the background of experience of the testees.

(14) The validity of a test—*i.e.*, the degree to which it fulfils its purpose—may be sometimes gauged by comparing the results of the test with the subsequent performance of the testees, in situations similar to, or different from, the test situation. But the more fundamental method of validation is the analysis of the mental processes evoked by the test, combined with statistical analysis of the factors probably generating the scores, this analysis being supplemented by comparison of the test results with any other information we may have about the testees.

If the contents of this chapter seem irrelevant to a book devoted, as this is, primarily to educational problems, it must be pointed out that refinement in testing and in the scientific interpretation of results is all to the good of education if it results in helping teachers to learn facts about the emotional and intellectual nature of their pupils, facts which can only be guessed by intuition and from observation in and out of school. It is true that the psychologist will pursue his way undeterred by considerations of the ultimate utility of his investigations, but that is no reason why teachers should not make what use they can of the results he obtains, when they have significance for education.

CHAPTER IV

EXAMINATIONS, OLD AND NEW

1. *Introductory*

THE vogue of " intelligence tests " presents a marked
contrast to the feeble and rather dismal kind of interest
that is commonly taken in " ordinary examinations ".   It
has generally been as objects of abuse that examinations
have occupied the public attention ; they are, in fact, the
constant butt of critics, who loose their bolts from many
directions.   Much of this criticism, being mainly destruc-
tive, soon becomes tiresome. The whole subject of
examining, however, broadly conceived as the art of
assessing minds by means of questions, is alive with
interest.

During the last fifty years examinations have, for
various reasons, developed to a remarkable extent.   They
have led to the building up of an elaborate machinery by
universities and other bodies, and there is no part of the
educational system into which they have not in some form
penetrated.   But the extensive and rapid development
of this machinery has been accompanied by comparatively
slow improvement in the examinations themselves.
Progress in educational ideas has indeed been reflected to
some extent in the type of question set, and examinations
have at times proved to be powerful instruments of
educational reform.   But if the examiner has the power
to lead education forward, he has also the power to hold
it back, and if the bad teacher often seeks to excuse his

weakness by accusing the examinations for which he has to prepare his pupils, the good teacher often finds examinations a real hindrance to educational progress.

There have been changes in the methods of examination, as distinct from changes in the type of question set, but these all belong to recent years, and have only been made by the more enlightened examining bodies. I refer chiefly to the endeavour to increase the reliability of examinations by statistically allowing for the unreliability of examiners. Criticism of examinations, however, has usually been directed against their syllabuses and questions, and the effects of these upon education, rather than against the validity of the examining process as a whole. But now that the growth of mental tests has drawn attention to the question of the validity of tests of ability, it is natural that we should explore that of the processes of gauging ability and knowledge by " ordinary examinations ".

As examinations have been in use for so long, and a large number of the people engaged in marking and setting the papers have been thoughtful people, it is to be expected that a good deal of valuable technique should have been developed. It is certain that much skill must be acquired by intelligent and careful examiners during their years of practice, even though the science that underlies their art remains a closed book to them, and to such people much of what follows may appear platitudinous. But if many mental testers have underestimated the complexity of their task, it is none the less true that some experienced examiners are inclined to overestimate the sureness with which they can perform theirs. There is no more difficult task in education than that of examining, and there are few more important. Oral and written examining is an essential part of teaching, and no teacher is competent in his craft until he has acquired much skill in interrogation.

2. *Aims of Examinations*

Examinations fall into several classes according to their aims. Thus, we have examinations that are primarily intended to test knowledge, and others that would be better called tests of skill. We have examinations that aim at the measurement of the actual attainment of the candidate, and others aiming at measurement of his capacity or promise. Again, some examinations purport to assess the effects of " general education ", whilst others, such as the qualifying examinations for various professions, have a more restricted scope and aim.

The purpose of an examination, like that of a mental test, is generally the measurement of an enduring or semi-permanent quality of the candidate. This quality may be knowledge or mental power, it may be something that is mainly acquired or something that is mainly inborn, it may be something of comparatively narrow range, such as the power to add numbers, or something of much wider range, such as the knowledge and ability in mathematics expected in a university honours candidate. But whatever the aim of the examination, our interpretation of the results will be subject to the principle of the single variable. The essay written by a candidate may tell us many things about his knowledge and his power, but if the essay receives a mark, we must at once ask, as in the case of mental tests, what single quality in the candidate's mind is represented by that mark ? What, we must ask ourselves, is the essential purpose of this examination, and does the mark give us the information we want ?

In examinations, as in mental tests, there is, besides the " primary indication " of the candidates' responses, a " wider indication ". In knowledge tests we can but *sample* the candidate's knowledge, and the wider indication of the examination is the total knowledge we infer that the candidate possesses. And the indication of many examinations is supposed to include mental qualities other than the actual knowledge sampled in the question paper. Indeed, if there is any justification for awarding university degrees or other distinctions on the basis of examination results, it must rest on the assumption that, when the candidates have forgotten most of the knowledge, and lost most of the specific skill, they evinced in the examination, something, " indicated " by the examination, remains.

But whilst it is generally the wider indication of an examination that chiefly interests us, the specific knowledge or skill it demands is sometimes our whole concern. Of a bank clerk, whom we have tested in arithmetic, we ask : Can this candidate calculate with accuracy ? If his accuracy does not reach the standard required in the banks, then the candidate must be rejected, and it is of no interest for us to know how the candidates who fail compare with one another in accuracy. Of a candidate for a navigator's certificate we ask : Can he find the altitude of the sun with a sextant, and so compute the ship's position ? If he cannot, then we cannot award him his certificate, however much ability and promise he may have shown. This dichotomy of candidates into those who pass and those who fail does not prevail in the domain of mental tests,[1] where we are interested in grading *all*

---

[1] This refers to passing or failing in a mental test *as a whole ;* in each *test item* the candidate usually either passes or fails (*i.e.*, he cannot, in any one item, show degrees of merit intermediate to passing and failing). And to serve practical, as distinct from psychological, purposes, it may

the candidates, however badly or well they may have done.

3. *Stages of the Examining Process*

In the examining process there are three stages, at each of which " ordinary examinations " differ in some respect from mental tests. There is first the designing of the questions, which, as it is fully considered further on, we can pass by here. Secondly, there is the answering of the examination paper. This may take several forms. The candidate may be required to write an essay or a series of essays ; he may be required to solve mathematical problems, or to design a machine, or to translate a passage from a foreign language ; he may be required to manipulate scientific apparatus with a view to solving a question put : but it would be idle to enumerate further the many kinds of activity through which we may put our candidates. A crude threefold classification of examinational activities is as follows : (1) We may ask the candidate—and there are many ways of doing this— to reproduce statements of fact, or of alleged fact. (2) Or, we may invite him to do some thinking, by interpreting facts, or solving problems, or in any way constructing and expressing ideas. Clearly (1) and (2) may be blended in an indefinite number of ways in any examination. (3) Thirdly, we may ask the candidate to give evidence of some form of skill, as when we set him an unseen passage for translation, or require him to take down in shorthand a dictated passage, or to add up a column of numbers. Here, again, there is no sharp line between (3) and (1) or (3) and (2). For, all skills, manual or

be useful to fix an arbitrary " pass-mark " even in " intelligence tests ", testees who fall below that mark being called " mentally defective ". The position of this mark on the scale will be decided entirely by practical considerations.

mental, involve knowledge of some facts, and thinking is itself a form of skill. In an examination in history, for example, a question will rarely call only for a statement of facts, but all questions will imply that the candidate knows some facts ; he may also be asked to interpret facts, which, if the interpretation is not a mere reproduction, will require thought ; and, unless the examination is very elementary, he may have to employ skill in the sifting of evidence and the putting together of his ideas into an intelligible piece of composition. Again, in a mathematical examination processes of all three of these roughly classified kinds—knowledge, thought, and skill—will be employed by the candidate.

The third stage of the examining process is the assessment and interpretation of the candidate's response. Here indeed we have a difficult topic, with which the rest of this chapter will be mainly concerned. A rough survey of the examiner's task shows that it varies considerably according to the type and aim of the examination, but that it has always two closely related aspects. The examiner has always (whether the examination products are essays, or solutions to mathematical problems, or drawings, or handicraft specimens, or musical performances, etc.) to assess the values of the candidates' *products*, and to arrive at a conclusion as to the candidates' *abilities*. A fine distinction, it may appear. But it is one that is often conveniently made. We may, for example, assess a candidate's essay on its intrinsic merits, and assign an ability, corresponding to our assessment, to the candidate. And in this case the assessment of the ability and that of the essay are virtually the same thing. But, on the other hand, we may assess the essay and then assert that, for a candidate of such an age, or who has had such and such opportunities, the essay is good, bad, or indifferent.

What is meant, when we say that an essay by a twelve-year-old pupil is good, is not usually that the *essay* is good, but that the promise of the *pupil* is high. Here, where our interpretation of a product is made in view of the age or other qualities of the candidate, there is a distinction between assessing the product and inferring the ability of the producer.

The most cursory review of the process of examining reveals certain problems of considerable difficulty. In the simplest kind of examining (such as that of an arithmetic paper which is marked for accuracy only) the examiner has merely to decide, a matter of no difficulty, whether a given answer is " right " or " wrong ". The marking of such an examination is, like that of a mental test, an automatic process calling for the exercise of little, if any, judgment. Few are the examiners, however, whose troubles end with so simple a task as that. Usually the examiner is faced with a set of products of a complex character, and in his assessment of any one of them has to take account of numerous aspects. And as the complexity of his task increases, so must the sureness of his judgment decrease. The problem at once arises, whether it is possible to simplify the process of examining without so simplifying the *candidate's* task that his product will cease to represent his ability. Or, the same problem may be expressed thus : where an examiner has a very difficult task to perform (as in the marking of an essay), it is unlikely that two or more examiners would assess the same set of products in exactly the same way ; what then can be done to increase the amount of agreement between examiners ?

One other problem may be mentioned here. It is usual to regard an examination as at one and the same time a measure of knowledge and of mental power. But examinations, like mental tests, are subject to the principle of the single variable. What is the way out of this dilemma ? How can we frame tests of knowledge that will also indicate mental power ? This question will be taken up in the next chapter. We turn first to the question of the agreement between the judgments of different examiners.

4. *Recent Criticism of Examinational Methods*

An examiner's judgment of the value of an essay, and his inference as to the ability of its writer, are both effects of very many causes. Some of these causes operate in all examiners who mark the essay, and, following the practice of writers on mental tests, we may say that such causes are "objective". Thus a candidate's statement of a *fact*, since a fact is something about which disagreement is impossible, is an objective cause of the examiner's judgment, if he is merely judging the correctness of the statement. Again, within certain limits of variation, the bare significance of the words used in the essay will be the same for all readers. According to the success with which the candidate can express his ideas, there will be more or less agreement as to the meaning of the essay as a whole—as to what the candidate is "driving at". But inasmuch as the candidate is unskilful in composition or confused in his ideas, there will be a certain amount of guess-work to be done by anybody who would gauge the mental qualities of the candidate by means of his essay. And where there is guess-work there enter into the interpretative process that goes on in the examiner's mind some elements that are peculiar to him. We may call such elements "subjective". The most obvious instance of a subjective factor is a bias against the candidate. Again, the examiner's "standard of marking", which may differ from those of other examiners, and may itself vary from time to time, and even from the marking of one essay to the marking of another in the same examination, is usually to a considerable extent subjective.

According to whether the determining causes of an examiner's judgment are objective or subjective, so we may call the judgment itself an objective or a subjective judgment. And so, if all examiners agree in making a certain judgment of the value of an essay, we may say that the judgment is perfectly objective ; if no two examiners agree, that the judgment is perfectly subjective. Clearly judgments can be arranged in an Objective-Subjective scale. Near one end of the scale would be such judgments as that the height of this man is five feet. Near the other end would be such judgments as that this shade of mauve is more pleasing than that shade. There is no such thing as an absolutely objective or an absolutely subjective judgment.[1] It is not possible to get perfect agreement even in physical measurements of " the same thing " made by different persons, but physical measurements are very highly objective. Nor would there be complete disagreement as a rule about the æsthetic qualities of a picture, but æsthetic judgments are usually highly subjective.

The ambition of the mental tester has always been to obtain results as indisputable as those of the physicist. It is natural, therefore, that he should gravely doubt the validity of a process so much less certain than physical measurement as the marking of an essay. And so enthusiasm for measurement in psychology has led to

[1] This is not strictly true. A statement I make about my own mental processes has wholly subjective causes (except inasmuch as I describe perceptions of objects that other people can also perceive).

criticism of the present methods of examination. Statistics have been produced to show that if a number of essays or other examination products are arranged in order of merit independently by several examiners there will sometimes be as many orders of merit as there are examiners, and that if any one examiner repeats after the lapse of time his marking of a set of examination products, there may be considerable differences between the orders of merit in which he places the products on the two occasions. This is a state of affairs that would never be tolerated in physics. A kind Nature makes it possible for all physicists to get practically the same result when, for example, they measure the density of iron. It should also be possible, say the critics of examinations, for all examiners to get the same result when they measure the density of Jones.

That objectivity is a quality to be secured in examining whenever possible cannot be denied. The critics, or " new examiners " as they have been called,[1] have devised forms of examination which are free from what they regard as the weaknesses of the " old " (i.e., the ordinary) examination, and which have what their authors regard as the cardinal virtue of objectivity. Only a few illustrations of this kind of examination can be given in this book. Before turning to these, let us seek for some of the causes of discrepancy between the judgments of different examiners.

---

[1] The reader who is not acquainted with the " new examination " will find it described with clearness, and (one might say) with gusto, in *The New Examiner* by P. B. Ballard. " New examinations " (or, as they are often termed, " Standard Tests ") have been designed for very many kinds of subject-matter in America. *Mental and Scholastic Tests*, by Cyril Burt, is a book that should be known to all teachers.

5. *Discrepancy between Examiners' Judgments*

There are several reasons why different examiners, assessing the value of the same examination products, or the abilities of the same candidates, are likely to differ to some extent in their judgments. In the marking of the simplest kind of answer, a statement of fact which is either correct or incorrect, no two competent examiners, it would seem, could disagree. But even here the examiner's *opinion* counts for something in his judgment of the candidate. Thus, whilst he must agree with all examiners in marking as correct or incorrect a statement giving the date of the Battle of Waterloo, he may differ from others as to the credit a candidate should receive for such statements as compared, for instance, with statements of opinion or attempts to interpret facts. And there may also be differences of opinion between examiners as to the completeness of factual statements that may reasonably be expected from the candidates.

In the assessment of a complex product, such as an essay, an examiner has to take account of many qualities, such as clearness of exposition, accuracy of factual statement, pertinence of argument, extent of knowledge shown, and so on. In order to arrive at a single mark for the essay the examiner must, consciously or subconsciously, arrange all these qualities in an order of importance, and allow them to influence the marking according to their position in this order. In his estimation of the relative importance of various qualities he will be guided by his conception of the purpose of the examination. Thus, in a test in arithmetic given to prospective bank clerks, the examiner may deem accuracy of calculation to be of more importance than power of solving problems, but in an examination (such as what is known in England as a Scholarship Examination) designed to single out gifted pupils for further education, the most highly valued quality in an arithmetic paper may be the power of problem-solving shown.   Now, examiners may well differ in their conception of the aim of an examination, and may differ accordingly in the relative values they attach to the various qualities of the essays or other products they are assessing.   One examiner may be much more influenced than another by a candidate's power of composition (in an examination that is not intended to be primarily a test of that quality) ; one examiner may highly value accuracy of detail, whilst a second is more disposed to credit what he calls grasp of the subject as a whole ; and whilst one examiner gauges a candidate mainly by the *conclusions* the candidate reaches (such as answers to arithmetical problems or interpretations of data in another subject), another examiner regards the candidate's *process of reasoning* as of the greatest importance, giving perhaps high marks to an ingenious way of reaching a wrong conclusion !

Examiners differ in several ways in their competence. If by conference a number of examiners define in detail the aim of an examination, and if in view of this they decide as elaborately as possible which qualities in a product shall be valued most highly, which less highly, and which shall receive no credit at all, and if these examiners then independently assess a number of examination products, there will still not in general be perfect agreement between their several assessments.   For, not all examiners have an equal power of discrimination between products with respect to any given quality ; nor are they equally capable of maintaining a uniform standard of marking. They differ also in their skill in the task, so often important and so often difficult, of " reading between the lines " of an ill-expressed answer, to form some idea of what the

G

candidate was trying to express. And there are other causes of individual differences in examining power with which we need not concern ourselves here.

Two distinct kinds of discrepancy, then, between the judgments of different examiners may be recognized : discrepancy due to their different *aims*, and discrepancy due to their different *competence*. If two examiners, in marking the same essay, give credit for different qualities, their assessments will not agree. But even if they are agreed as to what qualities should score most marks, they may still put different values upon the essay, for one may be more successful than the other in assessing any given quality. If Examiner A says that Candidate X is better than Candidate Y, and Examiner B says the opposite, we may ask, Which is right ? But we cannot answer that question until we are assured that both examiners were marking the essays from the same point of view. And then we have still to prefer one to the other. One man's word is not as good as another's. The " new examiner " believes that no man's word is any good at all.

If, it may be said, two examiners disagree as to the marks a candidate should receive, or as to the interpretation of the marks, they cannot both be right, although they may both be wrong. Disagreement between physicists as to the value of a measurement would be regarded as indicating one or other of two things : either that they were not measuring the same thing, or that one of them was measuring the thing erroneously. But examiners cannot agree so readily as physicists about what it is that they are measuring. As we have seen, even when the two examiners give the same mark to the candidate we cannot infer with certainty that they have made the same judgment, for they may not both have assigned the mark for the same reasons.

Where examiners have to judge *quality* (as distinct from mere correctness or incorrectness), such as the quality of prose written by a candidate, the merit of his method of solving a problem, the æsthetic value of his drawing, and so on, the process is bound to be to some extent subjective. The " new examiner " has attempted, with (he would admit) but little success, to devise objective methods for the evaluation of quality, in cases, such as the marking of essays or handwriting, where it is not possible to avoid judgments of quality. But in order to describe his proposals in this direction, we should have to make a statistical digression that would perhaps weary the reader and would be foreign to the purpose of the writer. In such subjects as arithmetic the new examiner avoids (at a price) qualitative judgments, such as judgment of merit of methods of working, by setting his tasks in such small doses (by composing his question paper of a large number of small questions) that any one dose can be taken by the candidate in one way only, and that way is either correct or incorrect. The only measure of " quality " he can obtain is the total number of these small questions correctly answered.

If we do not adopt the methods proposed by the new examiners (and in the subsequent Sections we shall see cause for rejecting many of their proposals), what can we do to increase the reliability of examiners ? In the first place, an examination is dependable only when it is designed and marked by persons who bear clearly in mind *the specific purpose of the examination*. Let the examiner be clear about what he wants the examination to tell him about the candidates. Do not let him be satisfied with such a vague aim as testing a candidate's " general education ", but let him ask further *what* effects of education are to be tested. Is he to look backwards to what the candidate has done, or forwards to what the candidate may be capable of achieving in the future ? Is the examination to test primarily knowledge attained or the attitude towards knowledge that the candidate's education has given him ? If the examiner has to set a paper in chemistry to pupils about to leave school, he must, in order to define clearly his aim, reach as clear an idea as possible of the part that chemistry can play in *general education.* If he misconceives this aim, and sets questions that are more suitable for practised chemists than for immature school pupils, then his marks, when included in a total (of the marks of many subjects), will impair that total as a measure of " general education ".

Examiners are no doubt to some extent, like artists, born rather than made. But to some extent also, like Londoners, they are made rather than born. Every inexperienced examiner should take his own making in hand. If he begins by attempting to mark essays to a finely graduated scale of qualities (giving, for example, any of the marks 1 to 100 to an essay), he should take steps to see whether such a fine discrimination is really within his powers. If he finds himself constantly giving low marks to candidates, he should suspect that he has not properly adjusted his standard to the general level of the candidates with whom, in his various examinations, he deals, or that he is not taking due account of the aims of the examinations. Above all he should, by careful introspection, study his mental processes when he is examining. His introspection will, like all introspections, be far from complete, but it will certainly lead to increased confidence and reliability.

6. *New Examinations for Old*

The " new examination " is an attempt to apply the methods of mental tests to the testing of knowledge, or of specific skill. The reader should compare the following brief summary of the methods of the new examiner with the statement of the principles of testing given in Section 9 of Chapter III.

The new examiner regards examining as a form of measurement, subject, like all measurement, to the principle of the single variable. His first step accordingly in the designing of an examination is to decide what quality he wants to measure. It may be knowledge of the geography of Europe, of the history of the United States, or of the principles of heat, and so on. He spares no pains in the task of ascertaining what are the " most important " facts in the field of learning with which his examination is concerned, and tries to draw up a series of questions that shall adequately sample the " essentials " of the subject. His next concern is to ensure that the candidates' responses to the questions shall be of a kind that can be marked in an objective manner. The candidate must not be required to write a series of essays in reply to the questions, for that would lead to error of measurement in several ways. If, says the new examiner, we wish to measure the candidate's knowledge of geography, we cannot at the same time measure his skill in English composition. Moreover, he may continue, power of composition is not even one of the determining factors of geographical knowledge, so that no credit should be given for skill, and no marks should be deducted for lack of skill, in the expression of such knowledge. And we have seen that it is not possible to secure high objectivity in the marking of essays. New examiners, therefore, avoid essays, or any other extended examination products, as they would the plague.   If the examining process is to be wholly objective, it must be virtually automatic, and the examiner's mind must be as far as possible eliminated.   The danger is lest, in designing our examinations so as to eliminate the mind of the examiner, we shall also eliminate the mind of the examinee.   There must be no judgment of quality to be made by the examiner; his but to mark as correct or as incorrect each item of the test.   Of the various devices that have been used to secure these conditions we can give only a few here.

Examples of " New Examinations " :—

(I) The " True-False " form.—A number of statements is given, and of each the candidate has to state whether it is true or false.

(1) The importance of Liverpool is due chiefly to its situation on the Atlantic seaboard.   True.   False. (The candidate underlines True or False.)

(2) To each of the following statements [1] the candidate answers " Yes " or " No," according to whether the statement is true or false :—

> (i) Boots are made at Stafford, partly because it is in the midst of a grazing district.
> (ii) The most ancient parts of London lie south of the Thames.

[1] From tests in *The New Examiner*, by Dr Ballard.   (i)-(v) from the test on " The Geography of England and Wales " ; (vi) and (vii) from the test on " History of England since the Accession of Henry VII (Tudor) ".   Tests (ii), (iii), (v), and (vi), as tests for use in class, are open to the objection that they bring false statements to the notice of the child, who is usually only too ready to receive suggestions, whether they are right or wrong.

(iii) The longest rivers flow mainly towards the west.

(iv) The most important mineral found in England is coal.

(v) All the great railway systems radiate from Birmingham.

(vi) James II was an ardent Protestant and tried to suppress the Roman Catholic religion.

(vii) In the first half of the nineteenth century slavery was abolished, punishment for crime was made more humane, and religious liberty was extended.

(II) The Multiple-Choice form.—A question or its equivalent is given, followed by several answers, from which the candidate has to choose the correct one.

(3) [1] " Write the number of the correct or best answer to each question in the parenthesis before the question ".

(i) ( ) Which city is nearest to Denver ?
<table>
<tr><td>1</td><td>2</td><td>3</td><td>4</td></tr>
<tr><td>Los Angeles,</td><td>Seattle,</td><td>St Louis,</td><td>Salt Lake City.</td></tr>
</table>

(ii) ( ) Which city has the greatest foreign trade ?
<table>
<tr><td>1</td><td>2</td><td>3</td><td>4</td></tr>
<tr><td>Buffalo,</td><td>New Orleans,</td><td>Augusta,</td><td>Washington.</td></tr>
</table>

(iii) ( ) Why are so many of the black race of Africa found in the United States ?

1. The people of the black race love to travel.

2. Most of them are not very industrious.

3. Their ancestors were brought here as slaves.

4. They are needed in the cotton fields.

[1] From a test on the Geography of the United States, by Buckingham and Stevenson (published in Bloomington, Illinois).

(4) [1] (   ) Wheat is grown in East Anglia because

　　1. The country there is flat.

　　2. There are no coal-fields in that area.

　　3. The climate is warm in summer and fairly dry.

　　4. The area is near London, which requires much wheat.

(III) The " Ebbinghaus " or " Incomplete Sentence " form.—The candidate has to supply the missing words in an incomplete sentence or group of sentences.

(5) " ——— is the chief wheat-growing region of England and Wales, because the climate of that region is ——— and is ——— in summer."

(IV) What might be called the " Multiple-Choice Ebbinghaus " form.—In each bracket the candidate underlines the word or phrase that makes the sentence true.

(6) " (Devonshire, East Anglia, Lancashire, Central Wales) is the chief wheat-growing region of England and Wales, because the climate of that region is (warm, cold, cold and dry, wet, warm in summer and dry)."

For the testing of bare information, especially if the candidates are young, and slow in composition, this form of examination has many merits.   It is usually an effective means of discovering what a candidate does *not* know, a discovery not always without value !   The marking of the examination is certainly objective, since there is only one way in which it can be done.   And since a candidate can answer a " new examination " question in one way only, there cannot, it might be supposed, be any ambiguity of indication.   For, on condition that there is no guessing of answers (and precautions, which need

---

[1] Tests (4), (5), and (6) have been devised as illustrations. They do not appear in any published test.

not be described here, are taken against this), we can certainly assume that correct answers indicate acquaintance with the facts demanded. There is often, however, as will presently be seen, a serious ambiguity in the indication of the " new examination ". The ambiguity may be described roughly as arising from the fact that a given statement, of the brief kind made in answers to " new examinations ", may be the object of various kinds and degrees of *meaning in the candidate's mind.*

A " Standard Test " is a test which is intended to measure, in an objective way, the attainment (in some form of skill or branch of knowledge) of a large group of children (such as all normal English or American school children). Such tests, in order to secure objectivity, are always constructed on the principles of the " new examination ". They are also—an important point— " tried out " on a large group of testees, the relative difficulty of the several items of the test, and the average score for pupils of various ages, being in this way determined. Tests of this kind have, in America, been constructed for all the subjects taught in schools. In England, Ballard and Burt have produced such tests for pupils in elementary schools, and a few have appeared in Scotland. The notion of an absolutely trustworthy examination, by which the attainments of the pupils in one school could be compared with those of pupils in any other school, and by which we could decide with but small risk of error whether any given pupil was deriving as much benefit from his school work as, in proportion to his natural capacity, he should, cannot fail to appeal to educationalists. If we fail to find such examinations we shall have cause for regret.

But can reliable tests of that kind be devised ? The answer at present seems to be as follows : For the testing of certain kinds or aspects of knowledge or skill the " new " examination is more serviceable than the " old ". In the testing of other kinds or aspects of knowledge the new examination fails, whilst the old examination approximately succeeds. Certain aspects of reading and arithmetic (but not the whole of either of these skills), lend themselves to " standard testing ". No doubt it will be possible also to devise " standard tests " that reliably measure certain aspects of other subjects ; but whilst the objectively testable aspects of other subjects are comparatively insignificant, those of reading and calculating are really important.

When we examine the standard tests that have been produced in such subjects as history, geography, science, mathematics, language and literature, many of us feel a pang of disappointment at the discovery we then make that what the tests can tell us about the character and extent of the testee's knowledge is so small in amount and so trivial in nature. We feel that many such tests aim at testing the wrong things. We should not regard the efficiency of our teaching as proved by the success of our pupils in these tests ; nor should we consider our teaching condemned by the fact that the showing of our pupils in some of the tests was poor. Reasons for the weakness of " new examinations " will appear in subsequent chapters, especially in Chapter VI. But one important reason may be mentioned here. It is that the " new examination " (or " standard test ") necessarily treats the knowledge of the testee as consisting of comparatively isolated fragments, whereas a candidate's knowledge of any one " item " is really an organic part of his knowledge as a whole. In other words, the piecemeal nature of the " new examination " renders it a less reliable instrument than the " old examination " for detecting the *meaning* the candidate's statements carry in his mind.

7. *Marks and Standards*

The usual practice in the marking of examination scripts is to credit the candidate with so many marks for each of his answers, and to regard his total performance as measured by the total of the marks for the separate questions. The examiner may employ a similar process in the marking of each question. He may divide the candidate's answer into so many parts, assess the value of each part as worth so many marks, and take the total of these marks for all the parts as the measure of the value of the whole answer to the question. Alternatively, he may for each question form a judgment of the value of the answer as a whole, a judgment which is not the sum of separate judgments of the parts of the answer. In this kind of synthetic judgment the examiner must without doubt take account of the various parts of the answer, or of its various aspects, but his judgment of the whole must be regarded rather as a single effect of his part-judgments than as their simple sum. And, whichever mode of procedure the examiner adopts, whether analytic or synthetic, he will, in most examinations, have to form some synthetic judgments : in the analytical mode he will have to judge the value of each of the *parts* or *aspects* of the answer synthetically.

There are doubtless very many causes contributing to such a complex act as the writing of an essay, but that fact is quite consistent with the possibility of those causes producing a single effect—the value of the essay as a whole, judged synthetically by " general impression ". Innumerable causes co-operate in making a man grow to his present stature, but that does not prevent us from obtaining a perfectly definite measure of his stature. Although the analysis of the process of synthetic assessment of the value of an essay, if it could be made, would be of great significance in the theory of examining, it would be absurd to suppose that " general impression " assessment must be relinquished until such analysis is forthcoming.

An essay has many diverse qualities. Let us, for a moment, compare the marking of an essay with the assessment of another kind of product which also has many aspects. We have to judge the value of a piece of woodwork, such as an ornamental bookshelf. There are several points to which we shall have to give especial attention if we want to arrive, by judging this specimen, at an estimation of the candidate's ability in woodwork. We shall consider the design of the article, how far it takes account of the purpose of a bookshelf. Thus if the distance between the shelves is so small that but few books could be found to fit, we shall put that on the debit side of the candidate's account. Is the design, we shall further ask, such as to produce a strong article ? Is it artistic ? Is it ingeniously simple or unnecessarily complicated ? Then we may turn to the workmanship. Does the article show adequate skill with tools ? Is the wood planed and sawn and chiselled with finish ? Are the several parts made to fit accurately, are they assembled carefully ? Now there seem to be two possible procedures for the examiner. He can maintain that every one of the aspects of the shelf (or the corresponding aspects of ability in woodwork) is important and should receive credit. He can say, This candidate shows very considerable skill in design, but is weak in the use of tools ; or, this candidate has mastered the use of such and such tools but is clumsy with others. He may continue by pointing out that, if he gives the candidate a high total mark because the design is excellent, he will be hiding the important fact that the workmanship is comparatively poor. The examiner will be saved from this difficulty, it would seem, only if ability in design and ability in workmanship always vary proportionately from candidate to candidate. And so the examiner may decide to give separate marks for each of the various qualities of the article ; he may avoid the invidious process of adding up these marks to form a grand and misleading total, and content himself with stating the marks for the several aspects separately. But there is an alternative procedure possible. Taking all the various abilities that are used in the making of a specimen of woodwork, the examiner may *estimate their relative importance*, mark them accordingly, and then take the total as an indication of the candidate's total ability. In this way he avoids any infringement of the principle of the single variable, for he obtains a measurement of the single thing—ability in woodwork as a whole. The validity of the process depends entirely upon whether there is a sense in which we can speak of " ability in woodwork as a whole ". For, upon the possession of a clear concept of that ability depends the process, mentioned above, of assessing the relative importance of its several components. All that has been said in this paragraph about the assessment of woodwork applies, *mutatis mutandis*, to the marking of essays.

The net result of any process of assessment is to place the examination products into classes. And as we always conceive these classes as having a linear order, it is often convenient to give them numerical names. Thus if we have nine classes of merit we may assign the marks 1, 2, . . . 9 respectively to products in the several classes. The marks then have the appearance of quantitative measures, but in truth they are only symbols of the classes into which the products are placed.

The standard of marking adopted by an examiner (by which we mean the scheme of assignment of marks to products of various merits) may be determined by what the candidates actually achieve as a group, or by what the examiner thinks they ought to achieve. In the first case the examiner is comparing the candidates with one another ; in the second, he is comparing the achievement of each candidate with a standard of achievement which is decided by the aim of the examination rather than by the actual level of attainment of the candidates. If we wish to grade a class of school pupils, and to select pupils for promotion to the next class, our chief interest will lie in comparing the candidates amongst themselves, rather than in comparing their attainments and abilities with, for instance, those of pupils in other schools. If we wish to select a number of pupils for the award of scholarships, we shall attain our end if we can arrange the candidates in an order of merit. But in such a case as this we should usually add, to the condition that scholarships were to be awarded to the top ten candidates (for instance), the condition that nobody was to receive a scholarship whose ability and attainment did not reach a certain level. That is to say, our standard would not be determined solely by the average attainment of the candidates, but also by our ideas of what the attainment of an individual should be in order that it should be wise to award him a scholarship. Again, in examining a group of applicants for certificates as air pilots, our task will not end with a statement of their relative merits. There is a minimum of skill which must be reached by any candidate before we can certify him as an air pilot. We may call a standard fixed, as in this example of the pilot's certificate, by the

aim of the examination, regardless of the level of ability
of the candidates, an "external standard"; whilst
a standard which is determined by the candidates' actual
performance may be called an "internal standard".
There is a determinable minimum of knowledge required
by a druggist, and that minimum is the "external
standard" fixing the pass-mark in a pharmaceutical
examination for the qualification of druggists. But even
in vocational qualifying examinations we have often to
fix the pass-mark below the real requirements of the
vocation, for, if the difficulty of the examination and the
position of the pass-mark were raised above a certain
level we should exclude more people from the vocation
than we could afford to do.

The meaning of this distinction between internal and
external standards will be evident if we consider the ways
in which the two kinds of standards affect the numerical
marks. Thus, we can choose our internal standard so
that the middle candidate gets fifty per cent. of the
maximum mark, and this it is often convenient to do.
But where there is an external standard in operation this
freedom is not possible. The external standard fixes
a *pass-mark*, and it is relative to that mark that we shall
mark the candidates. If the pass-mark is forty per cent.,
we obviously cannot give the middle candidate fifty per
cent. if more than half the candidates fail to reach the
pass-mark fixed by the external standard.

The practice of assigning $\alpha\beta\gamma$ grades to essays or
examination papers, especially to those of an advanced
nature, is very common amongst university teachers.
The method is favoured by some examiners because
numerical marks are wrongly regarded as necessarily
quantitative measures, whereas the judgments upon which
the merits of examination products are assessed are to

a considerable extent qualitative judgments. It is also often said by the advocates of this system of marking that, since their judgment is a judgment of the value of the product as a whole, it is misleading to represent it by a number ; for a number always has parts, and the suggestion conveyed by a numerical mark attached to an essay is that the parts of the number represent the values of the parts or aspects of the essay. The meaning of any one grade, such as a, varies to some extent from examiner to examiner, some regarding an a essay as a very rare thing, others assigning that mark more liberally. In this there is no difference between $a\,\beta\,\gamma$ marking and numerical marking. For, if the meaning of an a mark varies from examiner to examiner, so does the meaning of, say, eighty per cent. Nor is there any foundation for the claim, often made, that numerical marks are too precise for the crude process of assessing the merit of an essay ; for we are as free to limit the number of grades of merit when we are employing numerical marks as when we are assigning $a\,\beta\,\gamma$ grades.

In this chapter no attempt has been made to give a systematic critique of the theory of examinations. We have, so to speak, surveyed the shores of the subject, making a slight excursion inland here and there, observing the general lie of the land in some regions, leaving other regions altogether outside our purview. Some of the questions raised will be partially answered in the next chapter, in course of exploring the regions that we have hitherto left untouched.

CHAPTER V

THE TESTING OF KNOWLEDGE

1. *What is a Test of Knowledge ?*

" KNOWLEDGE " is one of those words that have a large wardrobe of meanings and are perhaps over fond of changing the dress or disguise in which they appear. Thus it has often been the custom, especially in books on education, to speak of " knowledge " and " skill " as though they were two different kinds of attainment ; yet, of a man who had skill in drawing, we should say that he knew how to draw and had knowledge of the principles of drawing ! Again, *knowledge* is often contrasted with *ability ;* yet knowledge of some kind is an essential component of every ability. A certain dictionary defines " knowledge " as " assured belief " and another dictionary defines it as " the clear and certain perception of truth and fact " ; yet these meanings cannot be regarded as the same except on the impossible assumption that what we believe with complete confidence is necessarily true. The second of these dictionaries also gives the definition : " Learning ; erudition ; illumination of mind ". Yet, excess of " learning " or " erudition " often renders " illumination " impossible.

This is no place for an excursion into orthology. But it is well, before discussing the testing of knowledge, to recognize that " knowledge ", " skill ", " belief " and " ability " are such closely allied qualities that no one of them can ever be considered in complete isolation from

H   113

the others. In particular we should observe that the
conventional dichotomy of tests into tests of knowledge
and tests of ability or capacity is crude, though certainly
convenient. The relations between knowledge and ability,
of which we must take cognizance in all attempts to
measure either ability or knowledge, raise some of the
cardinal problems of educational psychology.

Our immediate purpose is to decide what should be
included in the meaning of the phrase " testing of knowledge ". There are many kinds and degrees of knowledge ;
there are many components or accompaniments of knowledge, such as belief, attitude, and power. There is
knowledge that is best called " information ", and there
is the different kind of knowledge that is popularly called
a " grasp of principles ". The knowledge that the specific
gravity of, mercury is 13·6 is information; the understanding of the meaning of the term " specific gravity "
is knowledge of a different kind. But there is no clear
line between " mere information " and " understanding ".
If a boy can be said to " know " that the specific gravity
of mercury is 13·6, he must understand to some extent
what is meant by " specific gravity ". But the experience
of recalling the particular numerical fact about mercury
is clearly quite different from that of experiencing insight
into the concept of specific gravity. Constantly in
education and in testing knowledge we have to concern
ourselves with the interrelations between information and
understanding. And those are complex relations. Information about facts often promotes understanding of
principles ; whilst knowledge of principles is the frame-
work upon which most information is hung. In spite,
however, of the complicated interplay, in the process of
learning, between the acquirement of information and the
increase of understanding, it is not impossible in practice

to distinguish roughly between tests of information and tests of " knowledge of principles " or " understanding ". As a rule, the test of understanding has a wider " indication " than the test of information.

When we wish to devise a test of knowledge of a particular subject, such as history or mathematics, we have first to define more clearly our aim. We must ask, What do we understand by the term " knowledge of history ", as far as these particular candidates are concerned ? And the answer to this question will have at least two parts : the one part giving the range of information the candidates will be expected to have covered ; the other giving a statement of the kind of interpretation we expect the candidates to be able to put upon the information, the kind and amount of thinking about the information, the depth of understanding, of which we may suppose the candidates to be capable. There is knowledge and knowledge. There is knowledge that has been gained idly, the learner neither welcoming it nor, by taking thought, making it his own ; and there is knowledge which has been instrumental in strengthening the whole intellectual structure of the learner. There is knowledge that is only loosely organized, and knowledge highly and elaborately organized. There is knowledge which the learner has to a considerable extent, organized by thinking ; and other knowledge of which the organization was found ready-made in book or lecture. Again, there is knowledge of which the value, as a datum for judgment of the mental powers of a candidate, depends almost entirely upon how the candidate has come by it, whilst there is other knowledge of which all we ask is that the candidate should possess it, however he acquired it. There is knowledge which is held with some conviction by the candidate, and there is purely verbal

" knowledge," which is neither believed nor disbelieved. There is knowledge accepted upon authority by suggestion, and knowledge accepted upon authority with some insight into the value of the authority.

A test of knowledge, whether it be designed on the plan of the " new " examination or on that of the " old ", will aim at detecting some or all of the qualities of knowledge we have just mentioned, according to the particular aim of the examination. According to its aim, the test may be designed to indicate the extent of the candidate's information ; or the understanding the candidate has of the principles of a subject, and the sense which such understanding implies of the relative importance of various items of information. Other qualities that we may seek to test are : the character and degree of the organization of the knowledge ; the intensity and rationality with which the knowledge is believed, and the readiness with which it can be applied, by the candidate. Again, we may attempt to gauge, from the insight shown by the candidate's product, whether his knowledge is likely to endure or quickly to pass away. If our purpose is to ascertain the candidate's promise of further success in the kind of learning with which the examination is directly concerned, it may be important for us to know something of the manner in which the knowledge has been acquired : whether with ease or with difficulty, with strong or with weak " interest ", under the wing of a teacher expert in cramming, or more independently, with somewhat of the spirit of an original inquirer.

2. *Degrees of Understanding*

I have said that the word " knowledge " is fond of masquerading in many different garbs. It is generally considered that the most respectable of these is that of

Understanding, and the shabbiest Rote Memory. *" Sçavoir par cœur n'est pas sçavoir "*, wrote Montaigne, and almost all educational writers of note have said the same thing in other words. The dichotomy of learning processes, implied by Montaigne and the others, into " mechanical " processes, on the one hand, and " intelligent " or " insightful " processes, on the other, is but a crude analysis, slurring over, as it does, the most difficult of all the problems of educational psychology, that of the relation between habit and thought.[1] But though, as psychological knowledge increases, we may learn to speak more clearly about this matter, we are bound to recognize at once that the way in which knowledge is acquired, the attitude of the learner towards the knowledge, and the degree of insight with which he can contemplate what he has learnt, are essential factors of the value of his knowledge. It seems approximately true to say that knowledge adds to power to the extent to which power has been applied to the acquisition of the knowledge. And connected with this idea is the belief that much of the educative value' and powerfulness of knowledge acquired depends upon the kind and degree of the emotion accompanying or entering into the process of learning. " Learning by heart " is, according to this belief, the least educative mode of learning, because of all modes it has the least to do with the " heart ".

There are several senses in which we may speak of the degree or quality of a person's knowledge. We may refer to the number of items of which it is composed, or to the degree of organization of the knowledge ; we may refer to the intensity of conviction with which it is held, or to the clearness of insight with which it is appreciated.

---

[1] More strictly : the problem of the relation between reproductive and eductive mental processes.

Knowledge in the sense of a collection of separate items can generally be assessed with very fair accuracy by means of examinations. Degree of insight can often be tested indirectly by requiring the candidate to apply his knowledge to the solution of problems.[1]

Connected with insight is a quality that may be called the " potential " of the knowledge insightfully apprehended. The potential of an item of knowledge is its power of growth or of acquisition of further meaning. That London is the capital of England is a proposition of low potential; that God exists is a proposition of very high potential, for it may, in the mind of an individual, continually gain in richness of meaning. That the area of the square on the longest side of a right-angled triangle is equal to the sum of the areas of the squares on the two other sides[2] is a proposition of considerable potential, for it may be viewed from so many points of view, can enter as an essential factor into the solution of such a variety of problems, and can be " proved " (*i.e.*, rationally related to other beliefs) in so many diverse ways, that its meaning may continue for a long while to grow in the mind of the student. Examination products contain statements of various degrees of potential, a fact that throws the examiner on the horns of a dilemma. For, on the one hand, it is clear that the lower the potential of the statements evoked by examination questions, the narrower will be the indication of the candidates' answers. Thus the assertion by a candidate that London is the capital of England can have but small indication. As long as our tests call only for statements of low potential they can tell us comparatively little about the

---

[1] A " problem " may be defined as a situation the appropriate reaction to which must depend chiefly upon eductive mental processes, and only secondarily upon reproduction.

[2] The "Theorem of Pythagoras".

minds of the candidates. The indication of low potential statements is, however, generally without ambiguity. On the other hand, if a candidate makes many statements that have a high potential, the *possible* indication of his answers will be wide. In other words, the more meaning a candidate's statements have for him, the more would his statements tell us about his mind, *provided we knew how he interpreted them*. But it is generally extremely difficult to know how much understanding of a given matter is represented by a candidate's statements. Here, then, is the dilemma : the indication of low potential statements is narrow but certain, whilst that of high potential statements is wide but uncertain. The new examiner, believing in being certain about small matters rather than half assured about large matters, usually compels his testees to produce low potential statements of narrow but clear indication. The old examiner should accept the methods of the new examiner for what they are worth and as far as they go. But he should go further than that, with more uncertain steps no doubt, with neither undue confidence in his results nor undue scepticism as to the validity of his methods.

The problem of the measurement of degrees of understanding presents much difficulty to examiners, both old and new. This difficulty is due to two main causes. The first of these is the fact we have just mentioned, namely, that a candidate's statements often do not indicate clearly how much meaning they carry in the candidate's mind. This is especially evident in examinations in subjects of a highly abstract nature such as philosophy, or in subjects, such as psychology, in which terms are commonly used in more than one sense in different contexts and in which a problem of great difficulty has to be faced when we would give a clear definition of any given term. Teachers of such subjects often provide their pupils with an armoury of jargon against which the examiner, in his marking, has to fight at considerable risk of unfairness to the candidate. If a candidate asserts that " an instinct is an innate disposition which determines the organism to perceive any object of a certain class, and to experience in its presence a certain emotional excitement and an impulse to action which finds expression in a specific mode of behaviour in relation to that object ",[1] he may be saying something that has a considerable amount of meaning for him, much of which the examiner would approve as valid, or he may be saying something that means nothing to him, being reproduced without insight from a textbook or from notes taken down at a lecture ; or, again, the degree of his understanding may be anywhere between these two values. Taken by itself the candidate's statement has a very ambiguous indication. Whilst it is often possible to judge from the rest of the candidate's answer what credit he should receive for such a statement, this is by no means always true, and for that reason written tests in philosophy and psychology will continue to have serious weakness. The first source of difficulty, then, in the assessment of degree of understanding is the looseness of connection between thought and language, in consequence of which two or more candidates may use the same words without meaning the same thing. And the second source of difficulty is the plain fact that we need much more acquaintance with the psychology of understanding than is yet available before we can devise tests of understanding with a sure hand.

[1] W. M'Dougall, *An Outline of Psychology*, p. 110 (1923).

3. *Credit for Statements of Fact*

An important consequence of the fact that varying degrees of understanding may be experienced by a candidate when he writes his answers is that he should not always receive credit for a statement merely because it is true and is relevant to the answer. Even if he makes a true statement he may fail to understand it, or, if he believes it to be true, his belief may rest on erroneous grounds. This possibility of blind writing renders the examiner's task complex indeed. Sometimes the candidate saves his examiner the pain of doubt as to whether a given true statement is understood, by placing his gem in a setting of such obvious misunderstanding that its artificial nature, as an expression of the candidate's meaning, is at once evident. This is aptly illustrated by the story of the candidate who, when asked in a divinity examination at Oxford, " Who was the first king of Israel ? " promptly answered " Saul ". He was then allowed to depart but, wishing to make it quite clear that his knowledge did not end there, he added, as he reached the door, " He was afterwards called Paul." The fact that one part of a candidate's work may act as a commentary on another part, is one of the reasons why such extended answers as we obtain in the " old " examination are often so much more significant than the piecemeal answers of the " new " examination. At other times the examiner may feel inclined to refuse credit to a candidate whose answers smack too strongly of the textbooks he has read or the lectures he has attended, on the grounds that here is a case of " memory simulating other mental functions " ; the candidate, who should be thinking, is merely remembering—with what degree of understanding it may be quite impossible for the examiner to judge.

As a rule in such cases the examiner will have to give the candidate the benefit of the doubt ; he will have to assume that what the candidate says he says because he understands and believes it. But the examiner's treatment of matter that is obviously reproduced will depend to some extent upon the purpose of the examination. In an examination, for example, which is primarily intended to test knowledge of bare facts, we must certainly give credit for every true statement of fact. If the examination is an internal one, set by the examiner as a test at the end of a course of lectures (the usual practice in British universities), there will be no difficulty in discriminating between what the candidate has reproduced and what he has contributed as a result of his own thinking. In such a case, to the extent to which the purpose of the lectures was to convey certain information,[1] candidates must receive full credit for all true statements. But when, as is almost invariably the case, the lectures were intended to give understanding of principles, the examiner will not usually be content with answers consisting of quotations from his lectures, pieced together with more or less ingenuity. He runs, however, considerable risk of unfairness if he attempts to discredit true statements of facts or of principles on the grounds that he believes the candidate's understanding of them to be feeble. But if such attempts to judge understanding are dangerous, the examiner may legitimately and with

---

[1] As a rule no course of lectures should be concerned chiefly with the imparting of mere information ; nor is it generally either desirable or possible to test separately the information and the principles taught in the lectures. The content of lectures on *Materia Medica* would be mainly factual; but since all the information needed about *Materia Medica* could be found in books, there is little justification for lectures on the subject. Lectures to commercial students on office equipment and organization would be almost entirely informational. It is not easy to find examples of purely factual examinations.

safety exercise his art at another point of the examining process. He can set questions which cannot be adequately answered by reproduction alone.

If statements that are true should not always bring credit to a candidate, statements that are false should not always bring him discredit. If a candidate states that the fertility of north China is due to loess blown from the Gobi region, and the examiner regards this as an error,[1] the candidate should, at any rate in an elementary examination, be credited with having made a correct statement, as long as all the textbooks of geography with which we can expect the candidate to be acquainted explain the fertility of north China in this manner. In his assessment of error in any subject an examiner must take as his standard of truth the statements of authorities with which he may reasonably expect the candidates to be acquainted, and this standard will obviously vary with the level of difficulty of the examination.

4. *Words and Ideas*

Since in most examinations the candidate has to express his answer in words, any discussion of the theory of examining must contain some consideration of the interpretation of verbal expression. To some of the obstacles that stand between our reading of a candidate's words and our clear realization of his ideas we have already given attention. But what we have said so far on the matter refers to the interpretation of single statements rather than to that of a continuous piece of exposition. We have not yet adequately considered that most formidable of tasks, the interpretation and assessment of imperfectly expressed answers.

[1] See Rudmose Brown, Howarth & M'Farlane, *The Scope of School Geography*, p. 22.

The truisms about the inseparability of form and matter in composition, or about what is perfectly written having been perfectly thought, are of little service to the examiner, for he is dealing, as a rule, with the work of persons whose skill in thinking and skill in writing are immature and very imperfect. He has to give credit, where credit is due, for ideas that are incompletely expressed ; he has often to give credit for ideas that are incompletely formed. He has indeed to count clearness of thinking and of expression as virtues of a high order, but in so doing he must not leave out of reckoning qualities such as depth and breadth of thought which may be harder to assess. There are candidates who, especially when they are marked by inexperienced examiners, win by the skill of their pen marks that ought to be given only for skill in thinking, candidates who write so well that they get credit not only for the kind of clearness of mind that such facility certainly indicates, but also for originality, degree of insight, and other mental qualities that they may not in fact possess. One candidate's answer may be clear because he does not try to say much, whilst another candidate may, in a some-what confused answer, give signs, which a skilful examiner may interpret, that he is trying to say a great deal. It may be that, because he is trying to see so much further than the first candidate, the second candidate cannot see so clearly. It may be that some of the confusion of the second candidate's answer is due to his having perceived difficulties in the question of which the more facile writer was unaware. And, having read these difficulties into the question, the second candidate then adopts the plan, so serviceable to many people, in the examination room or in their own study, of " writing oneself clear ". A certain amount of such experimental composition is sure to occur in examination scripts, and where it does occur it may give us most significant information about the manner of working of the candidate's mind. We see, in such writing, a candidate's ideas in the making.

Are there not two kinds of confusion of mind that we may find behind an essay that lacks clearness ? Is there not, on the one hand, the confusion that is indicative of clearer and deeper understanding to come, and, on the other hand, the confusion which is a sign of permanent weakness of thinking power ? The first type of confusion of mind is comparable with the uncertainty with which a clear-sighted man observes a distant view, a view towards which he has the power of progressing, and of which in due course he will be able to describe the details, whilst the second type of confusion is to be compared with the imperfect observation of a man whose vision is defective. Amongst the most important and most difficult of the examiner's tasks is the relative assessment of answers which are confused through over-ambitious depth of thought, answers which are confused through weakness of thought, and answers which are clear because the writer has nothing ventured.

When a candidate does not *say* what he *means*, it may be because he does not know how to express his beliefs in words, or it may be because he does not know what he means ; that is to say, because his thinking is utterly confused. When a candidate possesses know-ledge that is largely of a " merely verbal " character, so that the words of the subject have but thin meanings for him, he may nevertheless manipulate words according to the rules governing the jargon of the subject, and so produce what may appear to be a highly creditable answer. In a written examination the extent to which a candidate's knowledge is " verbal " is often an unknown quantity, and for the detection of the degree of " verbality " of a candidate's knowledge the oral examination is a much more sensitive instrument than the written, where often a candidate does not *mean* what he *says*.

5. *Knowledge, Attitude, and Motives*

Jung has well said that " the first letter of the psychological alphabet is A for Attitude ". " Attitude " is a psychological term that we find easier to use than to define.[1] It is a word whose meaning, when it is used in everyday speech, is generally quite clear, and it carries practically the same meaning in everyday speech as it does in systematic psychology. The " attitude " of a student towards his studies is connected with the "interest" he takes in them, and with the intensity of conviction he experiences towards them. " Attitude " towards knowledge is also inseparably bound together with the value the student attaches to the knowledge. Not only, however, is the student's feeling that certain knowledge is worth while an essential factor of his attitude towards the knowledge, but his attitude largely determines the real value the knowledge has for him. The educative value of studies depends upon the student's attitude towards them more than upon any other factor, and it is therefore clearly important, especially when we are using tests of knowledge as indicators of " general education ", to ascertain as much as we can about a

[1] As a rough definition that will serve our purpose the following (from *Skill in Work and Play*, by T. H. Pear) may be accepted. " By ' attitude ' is implied all that we mean when we describe ourselves as being interested or bored, hopeful or despairing, excited or tranquil, serious or flippant." But the term is also popularly used to describe a general tendency to act in certain ways. Thus Pear writes that " one of the most valuable results of modern scientific education, when it is successful, is the cultivation of a certain attitude towards life which expresses itself in the habit of taking nothing for granted, except provisionally, if there is any chance of investigating its truth."

candidate's attitude. The opinions expressed by a candidate, when they are genuine, may to some extent reveal his attitude towards the field of knowledge with which the examination is concerned. But here again the oral test, applied by a skilful examiner, is more effective than the written. It is, moreover, certainly easier for a teacher to make a reliable judgment of the attitude of his pupils to their studies by observations carried over a long period than it is to test attitude by a single examination. This is one of many reasons for the keeping of full and systematic records of the mental progress of individual school pupils. If it is platitudinous to assert that teachers should be examining their pupils all the time they are teaching them, it is perhaps worth while to suggest that methods of making and recording observations of mental qualities should receive more consideration in courses of training for teachers than they do at present.

A great deal of examining must be conducted by written papers, and we have seen that attitude frequently fails to make itself clearly evident in such papers. The most important effect of this unavoidable disability of the written examination is the effect it may have upon education. For, if attitude, one of the main constituents of culture, can be assessed only in the crudest manner, examinations must be deemed very imperfect instruments for measuring the effects of education. It follows that they may encourage bad teaching by giving credit for knowledge that in fact contributes little to the culture of the examinee, knowledge imparted by teachers with small regard for the spirit in which it is learnt. And this effect of examinations is very evident at the present time. School pupils often " do " their physics and their chemistry, for example, in preparation for examinations, without ever experiencing the elation that should attend all discovery and scientific inquiry, and too often the knowledge they acquire is a burden of which they are glad to be relieved when they have carried it successfully through their examination. Those pupils who proceed to a university commonly obtain their degrees by a species of cramming differing from that of the schools only in being concerned with more advanced subject-matter. We should have to make a too wide (though an interesting) digression in order to consider the several causes of cramming amongst university students, but one cause, connected with the topic of " attitude ", may be mentioned. This cause is the excessive amount of technical knowledge that is demanded from degree candidates. It is often not possible for students, unless they have considerably more than average ability, to cover the syllabuses of their examinations and at the same time to maintain or develop that attitude of critical inquiry which is one of the aims of all education, elementary or advanced.

The uncertainty with which a candidate's attitude to his knowledge can be gauged in an examination is comparable with the lack of success that has attended the attempts of psychologists to devise tests for the measurement of tendencies and the detection of motives. The disability under which we are placed by the lack of adequate tests of tendencies and temperamental qualities becomes most evident when we wish to use test results as the basis of *prediction*. Tests of vocational fitness afford an illustration of this. An individual's fitness for a given vocation depends not only upon his ability, specific and general, not only upon his knowledge, but also upon whether he has, or may be expected to develop, a liking for the work, and has a temperament that will enable him to *use* his ability and knowledge. In the same way, if we would infer from the results of a candidate's performance in an " ordinary examination " the likelihood of his success in further study, or in activities not directly connected with the subject examined, it is important for us to know to what extent our examination touches what are popularly called his " interests ". In tests of knowledge it is usually an advantage if we can ascertain, what a candidate's script sometimes indicates, the motives under which he acquired the knowledge. There is clearly, for example, a difference between the indication of a piece of knowledge that was thrust upon the candidate and that of knowledge which he sought and found for himself. For, the knowledge which is sought in order to satisfy felt intellectual needs has more enduring effects upon the individual's mind than knowledge which meets with a less cordial welcome in the mind. This insistence upon the importance of knowing the motives by which a candidate has been impelled in his studies may seem to have a certain priggishness, inasmuch as it suggests that the disinterested pursuit of knowledge for its own sake is the only kind of study for which we should give candidates any credit. I do not wish to assert more, however, than that the *predictive interpretation* of examination results is much facilitated by knowledge of the various kinds and degrees of interest the candidate has experienced in connection with the subject examined, and of the sentiments that have been developed in the course of his studies.

In point of fact, of course, a student, when preparing for an examination, is actuated by a complex or hierarchy of motives, and the group of motives that may be loosely called " pursuit of knowledge for its own sake " is by no means the only worthy or important group. The desire to prove one's worth, to oneself and to others, and the pleasure of progressive achievement as such (*i.e.*, regardless of the special form of achievement, the particular

I

knowledge or skill gained), are, for example, motives that may healthily operate in the process of preparing for any examination. As incentives to work, examinations do not deserve all the censure that some educational enthusiasts have heaped upon them. Many students are guided and spurred in their studies by examinations ; many, including talented students, take considerable pleasure in planning their work in accordance with an examination syllabus. Yet no student, however uninspired and mercenary, ever works under the sole motive of passing an examination, for though, as more often than not is true, his prime motive is success in the examination, numerous secondary motives, such as interest in the solution of various problems, develop as his studies proceed.

It is not so much in the process of examining as in the construction of examination syllabuses that we have to take account of the importance of attitude in education. Since their power of influencing the work done in schools is so great, the examiners of school pupils (to take these examiners,[1] as the most numerous, for illustration) must base their syllabuses upon a careful consideration of the educational function of the subjects they examine. That should be their main concern. Whatever their subject they should consider what scope it should have, how much of its ground can be covered in school, *consistently with sound methods of teaching and learning*. This principle is, unfortunately, not always borne in mind by such examiners. Too often, in designing their syllabuses, they look forward to the work the pupil will do at a university (if he goes to one), rather than backward, to the work the pupil will have to do in preparation for the examination.

---

[1] British readers will observe that I have in mind the School Leaving, or School Certificate Examination taken by pupils at the end of their secondary school course.

Too often they consider what such pupils should know in order to profit by a university course (as such courses are at present), when they ought to consider what should be the starting-point of university work if the pupil is to reach it (by passing the examination) at a pace and in a manner consistent with the fullest development of his powers. And so they often produce heavy and wrongly conceived syllabuses which deleteriously affect the school work of both the ten per cent of pupils who proceed to a university and the ninety per cent who do not. There results a state of affairs in which much of the knowledge with which pupils leave school or enter university is, so to speak, known to them only by name, when it ought to be the object of an intimate and valued friendship.

6. *Knowledge and Ability*

" Ability ", like " knowledge " and all words, carries somewhat different meanings in different contexts, and it is important that examiners, when they speak of assessing " ability ", should realize as clearly as possible in which of its several meanings they are using the word. In common usage the term " ability " occurs in at least three senses which should be recognized as different from one another. It is used, especially in psychology, in the sense merely of " power to do ", regardless of the kind of task performed. Thus we may speak of ability to recall poetry, of ability to appreciate poetry, or of ability to compose poetry, three powers between which there are evidently marked psychological distinctions. Again, sometimes in psychology and usually in everyday speech, " ability " may have a meaning, which probably came to the reader's mind when he read the title of this Section, which may be roughly described as " the power to form new ideas, to apply knowledge to the solution of problems, or to react appropriately to novel situations ". In this sense, " ability " is in some respects contrasted with " knowledge ". When, in fact, we speak of a person as having " great ability ", we do not necessarily mean that he possesses much knowledge ; indeed we recognize that excess of " knowledge " may sometimes hinder the operation of " ability ".[1] But from the use of the term " ability " as meaning a power that, whilst it may employ knowledge, is itself distinct from knowledge, we easily pass, sometimes unawares, to a third use, quite distinct from the two others. We may, in fact, employ the word " ability " in the sense of *capacity*, a quality that is quite independent of knowledge and is possessed by the new-born, indeed by the unborn, infant.

The first of these three meanings need not detain us. The two others raise a number of difficult problems. They will lead us, if we let them, into that complicated discussion of the nature of " intelligence " and of " special aptitudes " with which many psychologists are now occupying themselves. But our purpose will be served if we only skirt that topic and observe some of the points at which it touches the practical task of the examiner.

In this matter of " ability " people are especially apt to make considerable assumptions, often without being aware that they are assuming more than is warranted by their experience. In an excellent old book,[2] for example, we read : " To discriminate between degrees of ability we must examine candidates in subjects which they have fully mastered ". Here it is obviously assumed that

[1] Somewhere (I quote from memory) Samuel Butler (of *Erewhon*) has written : " I do not know much, but if I knew a great deal less I should be much more powerful."

[2] *The Action of Examinations*, by Henry Latham (Cambridge, published in 1877).

" ability " is a general power, which may be applied to the study of various subjects. And the same idea underlies Dr Johnson's assertion to the effect that the important difference between two men consists not in the fact that one displays ability in, say, writing, and the other in fighting, but in that one has " more mind " than the other. But whilst this belief in a " general ability " is widespread, and has in fact some psychological sanction, people often use the term " ability " in a more restricted sense. They speak of " mathematical ability ", of " musical ability ", of " scientific ability ", and so on. And by " mathematical ability " (to take that example), they mean the power to think effectively about mathematical problems, rather than the possession of so much mathematical learning. At this point we meet a difficulty that runs deep in educational psychology. For, though we are all very ready to admit that knowledge and ability are two distinct things, we are bound to admit also that nobody can solve problems, nobody can adapt his thinking to novel situations, without knowledge and skill. Nobody can possess mathematical ability yet know no mathematics, though such a one may have great mathematical *capacity*, in the sense of potential ability. Are we, then, to suppose that mathematical knowledge is one of the components of mathematical ability? And if so, what is the other part of such ability? Is it " general ability ", which may function in any subject? Is it, on the contrary, a power of thinking which can only operate on mathematical materials? Or, again, is it a power of thinking which is in part general and in part specially mathematical? These are questions which can only be solved, and which psychologists are trying to solve, by empirical inquiry. But though these questions are as yet unsolved, the mathematical examiner is by no means entirely at a loss in his endeavour to gauge mathematical ability. For him, in fact, the question whether a person's power of thinking in mathematics is due to a general or to a special factor, is an academic one. For him the important thing is that he should know, not what are the deeper causes of success in mathematical thinking, but what are the mental processes that the mathematical thinker can observe going on when he solves problems. He must bear in mind, for example, that there is a significant difference between the answering of a question which is so stated that any candidate can at once see what principle or proposition must be applied, and the answering of a question which contains no hint of the lines along which a solution should be sought. He must bear in mind that the power to understand and reproduce, is quite different from the power to construct, a proof. Nor must he forget that, whilst mathematical thinking cannot be carried on without some skill in the manipulation of symbols, it is possible (indeed it is often desirable) to manipulate symbols with the exercise of very little (constructive or eductive) thought. These truisms, though they are apparently neglected by some examiners, are introduced here merely to indicate the lines along which the mathematical examiner must seek an understanding of the relations between knowledge and ability in his subject.

" Ability ", in the sense of power of constructive thinking, shows itself in different ways in different subjects. Every examiner has to consider what are the special signs of ability in his subject. In all subjects there are complicated relations between " knowledge " and " ability ", which vary according to the kind of data (*e.g.*, material things, as in science, or human records, as in history) with which the subject is concerned. There does not appear to be any useful general principle, applicable to all subjects, by which we may devise tests of ability, unless it be the following, which is suggested by the quotation we have made from Latham in the previous paragraph. In general, then, we may say that, the less a candidate is harassed by lack of information the more chance he has of showing ability. If, for example, in history, we set questions which make a heavy call upon the candidate's memory, we may be testing a power that is of the greatest service to an historian, but our examination will not be of a kind that is likely most effectively to test his ability. If in an examination in chemistry we set questions that cannot be answered without the reproduction of much detailed factual knowledge, we may or may not test the ability of those candidates who can remember such facts, but we shall learn nothing about the ability (which may be considerable) of other candidates to think effectively in the subject.

In this and the previous chapter we have reviewed certain principles that govern all examining. It is clear from what has been said that examining is an " art " that has a scientific basis which is but imperfectly understood. Hitherto the influence of psychological research upon examinations has been slight, and somewhat unhappy. But there is no doubt that as our knowledge of the examiner and the examinee, of learning and expression, of knowledge and ability, progresses, methods of examining will undergo great changes whose character cannot yet be foreseen.

CHAPTER VI

QUESTIONS IN THE MAKING

1. *Some Properties of Questions*

WE can leave to philosophers the task of fully analysing the nature of a " question ". They will find it a hard topic ; but it is the business of philosophers to find all topics hard. Discussion of any matter can always be conducted on one or another of several levels of abstractness, and the level we choose will depend partly upon the aim of our discussion. Our prime aim in this chapter is the furtherance of the practical art of interrogation, the art, that is to say, of inducing people to reveal their mental qualities through their answers to the questions we put to them. We are interested, therefore, in the psychological, rather than the logical, aspect of questions, in so far as those two aspects can be considered separately. We are interested in the effects our questions will have upon the minds they are designed to test, and in the interpretation of answers primarily as indicative of the mental qualities of the answerer. With this end in view we need consider only a few of the properties of questions, and that somewhat superficially.

From the psychological point of view, the most important property of a question is that it calls attention to a situation which is in some respect *incomplete*. The completing of the situation is called " answering " the question. From this simple principle we can deduce all the properties of questions which need concern us here.

Let us introduce an analogy.   Confronted with a circular arc we are at once able to think of the whole circle of which it is a part.   The arc may be a part of an infinite number of different figures, some closed, some open, some symmetrical, some irregular ; but our first impulse is to think of the arc as continued to form the simplest, closed, symmetrical figure, namely the whole circle, that can contain it as a part.   If, however, we are told that the arc represents half of a lens, the situation is changed at once, and although we may then complete the figure in one or other of several ways, drawing the complete circle will not be one of them.   If, again, we are told to construct a symmetrical geometrical design, of which the arc forms part, there is an infinite number of ways in which we may respond, and probably no two people would produce the same figure.

To what properties of questions are these of the circular arc analogous ?   First, before we can undertake to prolong it into any kind of figure, we must *think of the arc as incomplete*.   This thought implies *some* conception of the whole of which the arc is part.   We may think of that whole merely as " some closed figure ", or as " some figure obtained by prolonging the ends of the arc ", or as " some symmetrical figure of which the arc is the top " ; but it is not necessary at this stage to form an image of the whole figure.   Similarly, in order that we may appreciate a question as such, we must form some conception of the nature of the answer.   A question, in order to be intelligible, must to some extent define the theme and scope of its answer.   Hence the man who can ask, or interpret, a good question, is on his way to answering it, although he may know only the general direction in which the answer is to be sought.

Secondly, according to the instructions given, we have

greater or less choice in our method of extending the arc into a larger figure. Given that the arc is part of a circle, we can complete the circle in one way only ; given that it represents part of a lens we have considerable, but not unlimited, choice. Thus we may draw a convex lens or a concave lens, and in either case may exercise further choice in deciding what shall be the curvature of the other half. Given merely that the required figure is any symmetrical closed figure, there is no limit to the number of ways in which we may complete it. The fact illustrated in these examples, that we may have, according to instructions, various degrees of freedom in our task of completing the arc, is analogous to an important property of questions. The drawing of the complete circle is analogous to the answering of a question to which there is but one (correct) response. An instance of such a question is :

(1) *What was the date of the Battle of Waterloo ?*

To the drawing of the lens is analogous the answering of questions which, whilst they leave the answerer some freedom of choice of what he shall say in reply, yet confine his answer within somewhat narrow limits. Taking an example once more from history, we may cite the following as an illustration of such a question :—

(2) *What were the principal changes that took place in the government of a typical English village during the period 1756-1901 ?* [1]

And so we may pass to questions that allow great latitude to the answerer, such as :—

(3) *Show, by a discussion on any aspect of thought or of life, the essential unity of Western civilization.*

[1] I am indebted to Mr A. H. Dodd for assistance in the selection of several historical questions.

This property of the varying definiteness with which the answer is defined by the question is of such importance that we may conveniently give it a name. I shall call the degree to which the character of its answer is defined by a question the " *precision* " of the question. The question about the date of Waterloo has complete precision ; the question about Western civilization has very small precision.

Considering once again the problem of completing the arc, observe that the various ways of doing this differ in the kind and amount of insight they give us into the powers of the person who performs the task. The man who draws the complete circle reveals no more than an acquaintance with the simple properties of a circle, such an acquaintance as any normal person must form in the course of everyday life. The drawing of the lens shows knowledge of a more special nature, whilst in the making of the geometrical design considerable differences of inventive power may be revealed by different persons. We have already introduced the term " indication " to signify what a question tells us about the mind of the answerer. Since questions may have wide or narrow indication (compare the analogy of the arc), the reader will no doubt agree to the suggestion that the breadth or amount of a question's possible indication be referred to as its " indicative power ". An example of a question of small indicative power, in geography, is :—

(4) *Of what country is Vienna the capital ?*

Of greater indicative power is the question :—

(5) *Illustrate by a sketch map the position of Vienna as a focus of natural lines of communication.*[1]

[1] The objection to including such an example as this in a discussion of " questions ", on the grounds that it is not in interrogative form, is, of course, trivial. We might ask : What natural lines of communication lead to Vienna ? Or we might word the test interrogatively in several other ways.

Whilst the indicative power of a question such as the following is very considerable :—

> (6) *Describe, with examples, the various causes that may determine the site, and lead to the development, of a large town.*

2. *Precision of Questions*

Whilst a serious attempt at a theoretical discussion of the concept of " precision of questions " would take us too far afield, we ought here to consider somewhat more fully the bearing of the concept upon the practical problems of examining.   The new examiner always aims at designing questions of perfect precision, and his tests provide us with abundant examples of such questions. If the reader will refer to the specimens of new examination questions given in Section 6 of Chapter IV he will observe that every one of them is one-valued, in the sense of having only one correct answer.   It is clear that only by so framing the question that the answer consists of a single word, or one or two words, can we secure perfect precision ; for, if the candidates have to compose sentences in their answers we shall certainly not find that every candidate uses exactly the same words to express his meaning.   Nevertheless it is possible for two candidates to say virtually the same thing in different words.   If the differences between the *correct* answers to a question can only be merely verbal, the question may be regarded as, for all practical purposes, of perfect precision.   Examples of such questions are not hard to find.   Consider the following :—

> (7) *What natural regions are included in the State of Venezuela ?*

(8) *What are parallels of latitude and meridians of longitude ?*

(9) *How would you make a thermometer ?*

(10) *How would you prove that ordinary drinking water contains dissolved solid matter ?*

(11) *What are the properties that distinguish graphite in a marked degree from amorphous carbon, and what properties render graphite especially useful ?*

(12) *What was " Ship Money ", and by what famous man was it opposed ?*

The precision of every one of these questions is very high, although there might be differences of detail amongst the answers of different candidates. The details of the description of the process of evaporating drinking water may vary slightly from candidate to candidate, but the essential fact of evaporation will be mentioned by all who give a correct answer. According to his knowledge a candidate may introduce various facts relevant to the topic of Ship Money, in answer to the last of the above questions, but the essentials of his answer will be the same as those of any other answer that can be credited as correct.

It is evident that the greater the extent to which the essentials of the answer to a question are statements of " fact ", the more likely is the question to have a high degree of precision. But a moment's reflection upon the meaning of the phrase " facts relevant to the answer to a question " will reveal the following significant quality of precision : the quality, namely, that the precision of a question may depend upon the level of attainment of the candidates. In an elementary examination we ask :—

(13) *What were the causes of the French Revolution ?*

Applied to school pupils this is a question of fairly high precision, for since there is but little difference between the several accounts of the causes of the Revolution given in the elementary textbooks with which school pupils are familiar, all correct answers will be substantially the same as one another. But the same question in an advanced examination may produce a crop of answers between which there are essential differences. One candidate may stress the economic causes, another the influence of ideas ; one may show a considerable acquaintance with the original sources of the period, whilst another, less informed in that respect, may yet reveal more acumen in his critical discussion of the views of historians. In the advanced examination, then, the question has lost much of its precision, but—a point to which we shall presently return—it has gained enormously in indicative power.

Whilst, however, the precision of a question is often, as in the example just given, in inverse proportion to the general level of attainment of the questionees, this is by no means always true. Such questions as the following, though they may be answered more or less fully according to the knowledge of the candidates, are highly precise for any level of attainment ; the candidate has, in fact, little choice as to his method of treatment, and answers can only differ quantitatively :—

(14) *What natural regions are included in Siberia ?*

(15) *Trace the decline of the fortunes of the conspirators in* Julius Cæsar, *after Brutus' speech to the mob.*

(16) *How far did geographical features affect the problems of defence which confronted the Romans in Britain during the fourth century* A.D. *?*

(17) *What are the chemical properties of carbon dioxide ?*

Though candidates may differ in the amount of information they possess concerning carbon dioxide, their answers will have perfect precision in the sense that they will be either right or wrong, and in the sense that the factual field to which they are confined (namely, the properties of carbon dioxide) is defined by the question. Of somewhat less precision are questions that give the candidate some choice in his response, in as much as he can choose, within certain limits, the subject-matter about which he writes, but which call for answers of a factual nature that are either right or wrong. For example :—

(18) *Name a country in which the climate is hot and damp, and state what are the chief products of the region and the occupations of the people.*

(19) *Give examples of* (a) *a good harbour with a productive and accessible hinterland ;* (b) *a good harbour with an unproductive hinterland.*

(20) *Mention examples of each of the following varieties of metallic oxides :* (a) *readily soluble in water ;* (b) *slightly soluble in water ;* (c) *insoluble in water.*

Before we conclude these examples of questions of various degrees of precision mention must be made of a class which includes some of the best and some of the worst questions. I refer to questions that require the candidate to express an *opinion*, in the sense of a judgment based upon incomplete data. Since *no* judgments (except possibly those made in pure mathematics) are completely justified by the data upon which they are based, it is clear that all judgments have an element of opinion in them. But in some matters the element of uncertainty is so large that men must differ considerably in their judgments concerning them, and we then find, and are content to find, that " opinions differ ". Thus a man may claim that, " in his opinion ", Beethoven's Seventh Symphony is better then his Eighth, though Beethoven himself (whether or not he meant what he said) expressed the reverse opinion.[1] Or, again, two men may hold opposite opinions as to the possibility of abolishing war between civilized communities. Suppose, to bring the topic of " opinion " into relation with the problems of examining, that this question is put to a class of university students :—

> (21) *What is your opinion as to the possibility of abolishing war amongst civilized peoples ?*

Here indeed is an excellent example of a question of low precision, for there will certainly be great differences between the answers given by different candidates. How is the value of a candidate's answer to this question to be assessed ? The question I have just written—as to the mode of assessment of candidates' answers—would no doubt itself give rise to differences of opinion amongst examiners. On the mode of assessing candidates' opinions examiners should try to agree, but it would be a mistake to wait until all examiners were agreed on this matter, before we ventured to introduce such questions as (21) into examination papers. A candidate may, of course, reveal various degrees of knowledge of international affairs, and various degrees of acumen in his discussion of them, whether he declares for the possibility of abolishing war or for the opposite view. He may also reveal bias of

---

[1] It may be claimed that, in the realm of value, we ought not to expect agreement, even between competent persons ; that, in short, " taste " cannot have objective validity. If then a candidate preferred *Casabianca* to the *Ode to the West Wind* we should have to accept his judgment as " valid for him ", provided that it was sincere. But we should certainly deplore it, a fact that seems to indicate that æsthetic values have a certain objectivity.

various kinds and degrees. And the conclusion at which the candidate arrives may or may not agree with the opinion the examiner himself holds. Of statements of fact concerning international affairs the examiner can without difficulty judge the value ; of the candidate's power of thinking, the logical coherence of his argument is a clear indication, provided the examiner knows that the argument is not a mere reproduction. Of " bias " the examiner may be able to distinguish between two kinds : on the one hand, the bias that is unthinkingly taken over from authority, on the other hand, bias that is the emotional expression of a sincere attempt to think and act rightly in the complicated situations of human life. The value of the candidate's opinion must then be judged according to its consistency with the evidence he cites in support of it, according to the adequacy and validity of the evidence itself, and according to the sincerity of conviction with which the opinion appears to be held. And in judging the adequacy and validity of the evidence, the examiner must, of course, take account of the limitations of knowledge that must necessarily hinder candidates of such and such an age or experience. Disagreement of opinion between the candidate and the examiner, as to the possibility of ending war, should not necessarily adversely affect the examiner's assessment of the candidate's answer. The examiner, in fact, is not to judge the value of the candidate's opinion as an opinion sanctioned by his (the examiner's) knowledge and experience, but as sanctioned by the knowledge and experience of the candidate.

The considerations given in the last paragraph apply *mutatis mutandis* to such " opinion questions " as the following :—

(22) " *Human progress is little more than a surplus of*

K

*advantages over evils ". Discuss this dictum in
reference to the social results of the Industrial
Revolution.*

(23) *What is your opinion of Oliver Cromwell as a man ?*

(24) *Which of the following do you consider to have done
the greatest work for the development of the British
Empire : Lord Durham, Cecil Rhodes, Lord Cromer ?
Give reasons for your answer.*

Occasionally an examiner will word a question as
though it demanded an opinion when the answer to the
question is purely factual. This practice, which, though
it is undesirable, seldom gives rise to ambiguity in the
question, is illustrated by the following :—

(25) *What do you consider* (a) *two of the most densely
populated, and* (b) *two of the least populated, parts
of the United States ? Account briefly for the facts
in each case.*

The phrase " what do you consider " suggests that the
density of population of parts of the United States is
a matter of opinion.

Since the precision of a question, set for a given group
of candidates, depends chiefly upon the amount of knowledge they have relevant to the question, being generally
small when that knowledge is large, and *vice versa*, it is
easier to set highly precise questions in elementary than
in more advanced examinations. This is one reason why
the new examiner, whilst he has met with some success
in the testing of knowledge at an elementary stage, fails
completely when he attempts to deal with more advanced
stages. For, the essential quality of questions in new
examinations is that they are absolutely precise.

3. *Indication of Questions*

The " precision " of a question is the extent to which the answer is defined by the question ; or, what amounts to the same thing, the limits within which a candidate's answer must lie if he is to score credit for it. A question of perfect precision compels the candidate to run, so to speak, on a single line of rails, whilst a question of low precision, though it defines the region in which he must move, leaves him free to follow any path in that region he may choose. Very often the more freedom we give a candidate the more opportunity we give him of showing his powers. All questions must, however, make clear to the intelligent candidate the general direction in which his answer should run. A question must set a definite problem, though it may be a problem that may be approached in several different ways. According to his aim the examiner will set a question of high or low precision. If, for example, he wishes to test the candidates' knowledge of the positions of certain places on a map of France, he may not rest content with such a question as :—

(26) *On a sketch map of France show the positions of the chief towns,*

but may prefer to set one or other of the following :—

(27) *On a sketch map of France mark the positions of Paris, Lyons, Marseilles, St Etienne, Bordeaux, Calais, and Havre ;* or

(28) *What are the names of the towns whose positions are represented by the numbered dots on the map provided ?*

Questions (27) and (28) are more definite and easier to mark fairly than question (26). The indication of these last two questions is clearer than that of the first, since if a candidate omits, say, Lyons, from his answer to (26), we cannot conclude that he does not know where that town is situated. On the other hand, question (26) gives the candidate a chance of showing more knowledge than he can show in answer to either of the two other questions. The precision of (26) is lower than that of the other questions, but whilst its *possible* indication is higher, it does not indicate without ambiguity what we want to know about the candidate—whether, in short, he can locate certain places. This is in conformity with the principle which, we have seen, usually holds good, that the narrower the desired indication, the higher should be the precision of the question.

The examiner, like the mental tester, must be guided in his design of a question by as clear an idea as possible of what he wants the question to tell him about the candidate. And to test a particular ability, or the understanding of a particular principle, he will have to frame questions that will give all candidates who possess that ability or understanding the best chance of showing it. A question should often not only put a problem to the candidate, but should also give him some guidance towards its solution. Compare, for example, the following two questions :—

(29) *What causes determine the boundaries between states ? Give examples of the different kinds of boundaries, and explain why, in the instances you give, one kind of boundary rather than another was chosen.*

(30) [1] *On an outline map of the United States, colour all the boundaries, both state and national, according to the following scheme : (a) boundaries determined by*

---

[1] From *Principles of Human Geography*, by Huntingdon and Cushing (New York, 1922).

mountains—red ; (b) *by water—blue ;* (c) *by deserts —yellow ;* (d) *by arbitrary lines of latitude and longitude or other straight lines—green. Discuss your map to show what parts of the country are characterized by each kind of boundary, and why ?*

In many respects question (29) is harder than question (30). But much of its difficulty is of a kind that *hinders* the candidate from revealing his understanding, which may be considerable, of the principles to which the question refers. For, in answering (29) he has to *recall* examples of boundaries, a feat of memory which has no connection with the desired indication of the question, which is an understanding of certain geographical principles. Question (30) is therefore the better of the two. It is of greater precision than the other question, but it is of more certain indication.

It is often well to increase the definiteness of the indication of a candidate's answer by clearly defining the lines he must follow, as is done in question (30). Questions whose precision is increased by clauses controlling the candidate's answer, but which yet leave him much scope, are often the most effective means of testing understanding of principles. Such questions deserve a wider use. Though the following question is unconscionably long, and perhaps too generous in the help it gives the answerer, it is worth quoting in full :—

(31) [1] *The international relationships of China are unique. This is partly a matter of racial character and historical development, but geographical conditions enter into it. Describe these conditions and their international results. Among other things consider the following :* (a) *the effect of density of population*

[1] Huntingdon and Cushing, *op. cit.*

on China's prosperity at home and on foreign trade;
(b) China's degree of geographic diversity or uni-
formity, and its effect on both internal and external
trade; (c) the boundaries of China and their effect
on international relations; (d) the relatively inert
character of the Chinese; (e) the position of Japan
relative to that of other energetic nations; (f) the
energy of Japan relative to that of other Asiatic
nations; (g) the resources of China; (h) the accessi-
bility of the Chinese coast and of the interior, and the
development of transportation.

When the prime aim of a question is to test understanding of principles, the effectiveness of the question
increases with every precaution we take against the
candidate's being able to answer by reproduction of
memorized material. A question demanding a mere
definition of a principle produces answers whose indication
is indefinite because it is not possible for the examiner to
judge with what degree of understanding they are written.
By asking the candidate to give examples of the validity
of the principle we improve the question slightly, but the
question is still an imperfect test of understanding. For,
the candidate's illustrations may be those provided by
textbook or teacher, and he may understand them no
better than he understands the principle itself. Let us
put the question

(32) *State Newton's Third Law of Motion and illustrate*
its meaning by examples.

Few can fail to remember the words "Action and
reaction are equal and opposite", but many can fail to
understand them. Nor does a candidate prove his understanding by quoting the illustrations in vogue in textbooks
of mechanics: such as, that when a book rests upon a table,

the table pushes the book up with a force equal to that with which the book pushes the table down. The weak candidate, who cites a tug-of-war as an illustration of the law, may often cherish a secret belief that " in reality " the winning side applies a somewhat greater force *to the rope* than does the losing side. But if he wisely refrains from mentioning this belief he may earn credit for understanding the law although he is evidently in a state of the utmost confusion about it. The most reliable indication of understanding of such a principle as Newton's Third Law will be supplied, in an elementary examination, by questions which require the candidate to apply it to the solution of problems he has not seen before. In an advanced examination, on the other hand, the candidate might be asked to write a critical account of the logical basis on which the statement of the law rests.

4. *Suggestion and Guidance in Questions*

The object of a question is to initiate thought or the reproduction of ideas. That questions may differ in the definiteness with which they perform this function, some evoking a specific reproduction, others starting a train of thought and reproduction which may vary much from candidate to candidate, is abundantly illustrated in the previous two Sections. The definiteness with which a question suggests its answer depends upon its wording and upon the state of the candidate's mind, including his knowledge and past experience. In continuation of the foregoing discussion we may here point out a distinction which is of some consequence in the theory of interrogation, a distinction which, in fact, examiners rarely fail to make in practice. I refer to the discrimination of three classes of questions : those, namely, that tell the candidate

too much, those that tell him too little, and those that
tell him just as much as is necessary to ensure that his
answer will have the desired indication. A trivial example
of a question which tells too much, quoted from a
" scholarship paper " for elementary school pupils is

(33) *Can a place on the Equator be cold ? Why not ?*

Here the wording of the first part of the question suggests
the answer " No " ; but for fear lest the suggestion should
not be strong enough, the examiner obligingly gives his
candidates an unmistakable answer to the first part of
his question by adding the laconic " Why not " ? He
would have tested the candidate's knowledge equally
well, and have avoided silliness, if he had asked

(34) *Why are places near the Equator hotter than other
parts of the world ?*

Some questions are so strongly suggestive that they
amount practically to a positive assertion. Thus

(35) *If you are so ill, would it be wise to run in the race ?*

would generally be spoken, not as a question proper, but
merely as an interrogative form of the statement " You
are too ill to run safely in the race ".

Questions that tell the candidate too little are exemplified
by those which, while they are intended primarily to test
the candidate's understanding of a principle, demand the
reproduction of much knowledge that a candidate who
fully understands the principle may not have at his beck
and call. Question (29), on the boundaries of states, is
a question of this kind. Questions of this kind are
occasionally set in mathematics, problems being set that
can be solved only if the candidate remembers a formula,
although the power to recall the formula is irrelevant to
the chief indication of the question. If, for example,

a question whose solution includes finding the volume of a sphere (such as question (36) below), is set in an *elementary* examination, it may be advisable to supply the candidate with the formula for the volume, since, at an elementary stage of study, it is not important that the pupil should carry such formulæ in his head, whilst it is important that he should know how to *apply* them :

(36) *The gas-bag of an airship consists of a cylinder 180 feet long, of diameter 60 feet, with a hemisphere at each end. How many cubic feet of gas can it contain ? A sphere of radius* r *has a volume* $= \frac{4}{3}\pi r^3$.

In deciding how much information he shall give the candidate, or how much guidance by controlling clauses (see Section 3 above), the examiner will, of course, be guided principally by the indication he wants the candidate's answers to have. His chief aim in setting question (36) is to test the candidate's power of dealing with the volumes of such compound solids as the sausage-shaped gas-bag, but if he omits to provide the formula, he will clearly fail to test that power in a candidate who does not happen to remember the formula.

5. *The Ease of being Difficult*

It is easy for an examiner to set questions that he himself cannot answer. It is also easy for him to set questions that he can answer, but which would have been beyond his powers a week before he set the paper. In a happy moment, we will suppose, an examiner invents (or discovers in a book) the following neat geometrical construction for finding the reciprocal of a number. OO′ is one inch long and a circle is drawn with OO′ as

a diameter. Draw tangents OT, O'T', at O, O' respectively, T and T' both being on the same side of OO'. To
find the reciprocal of any number, x, take a point, X, in
OT, such that OX is x units long. Join XO', cutting
the circle in S. Draw OS, and produce to cut O'T' in
X'. Then the number of inches in O'X' is the reciprocal
of x. (If the reader will sketch a figure according to these
instructions he will find that it is an extremely simple
construction. Descriptions of geometrical constructions
have, in order to avoid ambiguity, to be given in a detailed
form that makes them seem complicated to the person
unfamiliar with mathematics.) Now suppose that the
examiner sets the question :—

(37) *Give a geometrical construction for finding the
reciprocal of any number.*

Unless the construction the examiner has in mind, or
some other construction, for finding reciprocals, is common
knowledge which all young pupils may be expected to
possess, question (37) is an extremely difficult one. Few
candidates, if any, in an advanced university examination
would succeed in *inventing* the construction we have
described above. If the examiner, when he is considering
the suitability of question (37), will imagine himself
confronted by that question, without any previous
knowledge of the method of solution, he may conclude
that he, at least, would probably fail to answer it. If,
however, he wishes to frame a question on the construction
for an elementary examination, he can fairly do so by
stating the construction in the question and merely
asking the candidate to prove it. This mathematical
example illustrates the obligation under which all
examiners, in all subjects, lie, of attempting to answer
their own questions, *from the point of view of the candidate,*

(*who does not already know the answer*), before they include the questions in an examination paper.

Inexperienced examiners often set unduly hard papers because they mistake their purpose. They forget that their purpose is generally to give candidates the maximum opportunity of showing their mettle, and that, therefore, excessively hard papers are as ineffective as excessively easy papers. Though most of their candidates are geese, such examiners set a paper fit only for swans, on the plea that, if the geese are not swans, they ought to be. They pay less attention, when designing their questions, to what their candidates are likely to be able effectively to do, than to what they (the examiners) think the candidates " ought " to be able to do. And if, as is often the case, the young examiner is of above average ability, he is apt to think that candidates " ought " also to be above the average. In this way he sets " unfair " questions. A "fair" question is one which evokes answers that really indicate the qualities that the examination is intended to test.

The questions so far considered have been those of written examinations. The design of such questions, so that they shall unambiguously present the problem the examiner intends the candidate to solve, and shall produce answers that may be assessed with reasonable accuracy, is a task, full of difficulty, which the young examiner should assume that he only imperfectly understands. Always the examiner in a written examination must to some extent *guess* what effects his questions will have upon the candidates. But guessing is a mental process that may be of no mean order ; it is a process, in fact, that all thinkers and inquirers have continually to use. There are good guessers and bad guessers. Learning to think consists largely in learning to guess well. At the beginning of their examining careers, examiners should regard themselves as serving a period of apprenticeship in which, by critical observation of their methods, combined with a study of such aspects of the theory of examining as are described in this book, they acquire, amongst other skills, that most valuable element in the examiner's art, the power of intuitively judging, of wisely guessing, the significance of the candidate's written word.

But this chapter would end on a false note if the foregoing eulogy of guessing were not qualified. Practitioners in any art are too ready to extol intuition and to assume that reliable intuitions will come to him who only waits for them. There is no lack of teachers, for example, who regard educational research as a clumsy attempt to solve problems that "the good teacher solves by intuition". There is no lack of examiners who suppose that, because examining is an art, attempts to formulate principles of examining, with due regard to the latest relevant findings of psychology, are ill-advised and unnecessary. The reliability of an examiner's intuitive judgments depends, however, to a great extent upon the amount of thought he has given to the principles underlying his art. The examiner's attempts of yesterday to think clearly about the principles of examining may lead to more reliable intuitions to-day, and the intuitions of to-day provide the material for the principles of to-morrow.

CHAPTER VII

QUESTIONING IN THE CLASSROOM

1. *Introductory*

PRECEPT cannot anticipate all the conditions that may confront a teacher in the classroom, all the procedures the inspiration of the teacher may produce or the behaviour of the pupil may suggest. Nor is it possible to describe with exactness all the qualities of the teacher who is master of his craft. Hence all writings on teaching suffer from an incurable weakness. But they are not therefore unnecessary. That an amateur actor should be told to face the audience as much as possible is not proved to be unnecessary or misleading advice by the fact that the back of a skilled actor may often be eloquent. That the amateur had better try to follow many general rules is good advice, not rendered idle by the fact that many good actors break many of the rules. So, there is needed no apology for rules of procedure given to young teachers, provided that the rules are sufficiently elastic, are based upon experience of teaching, and are not forced upon the teacher, without regard to his individual nature, in a way that renders him less effective than he would be without them.[1] There are many details of questioning, such as the tone of voice, the manner and expression of the teacher, which, capable as they are of infinite variation,

---

[1] Considerable tact has to be exercised by trainers of teachers in order to ensure that, whilst advice is given when it is needed, the individuality of the teacher is duly considered at every point of the training process.

cannot be adequately described, and must be left to the initiative of the teacher and to the practical skill and tact of those who attempt to train him. Yet, there is no more interesting, no more important or difficult, branch of the teacher's art than that of asking questions, and this is a matter in which the trainer of teachers can render very valuable and immediate service to his students.

A " question ", says a dictionary, is " a seeking : an inquiry : an examination, especially by torture ". The last of these three definitions best describes the questions we have considered in the foregoing chapters. We have considered questions as *tests*. In the present chapter we shall be mainly concerned with other aspects of questioning. The question may be used in many ways as part of the process of teaching. It may be used to test the effects of previous teaching, and this use has several aspects. Thus it helps to form or confirm the teacher's opinion of the abilities of his pupils ; it indicates the effectiveness of the methods he has employed, and may help to decide the methods he will employ in subsequent work. The question as a test has also usually to be employed as a preliminary to the introduction of a new topic, indicating as it does the pupils' background of knowledge, acquired in or out of school, which the teacher has to consider in deciding his method of leading up to the topic. The main value of such questioning lies perhaps in its determination of the part the *pupils* can play in the lesson in which the new topic is developed ; how much can they, in their answers to further judiciously chosen questions, contribute to the development ? The asking of a series of questions is often the best way to induce pupils to make an intuitive judgment, which will be confirmed or rejected in the course of the lesson. And allied to this *rôle* of questions is the part they may play in arousing interest, and in initiating trains of associated ideas and of reasoning which lead in the direction of the topic to be introduced. Questions of this kind will often be questions that none of the pupils can answer at the time they are asked. Thus we may ask a class of beginners in science whether the moisture observed on windows in cold weather is on the inside or the outside of the window, a question that some, but probably not all, of the pupils will be able to answer ; and we may next ask why the moisture is there at all. We do not ask this last question because we want to discover whether the pupils know the answer. We ask it because we know that they do not know the answer ; we ask it in order to call attention to the phenomenon, to present the moisture on the windows as an *incomplete situation* which the pupils will then desire to complete ; that is to say, having been induced by the question to regard the moisture on windows as an unexplained fact, they will wish to know the explanation. The aim of such a question as this about windows may be regarded as the creation of a state of doubt in a matter concerning which the pupil had no doubt before. This creation of *productive* doubt (there are some kinds of doubt that it is unwise to induce in the pupil's mind) is a common use of questions in teaching. Mathematics provides innumerable examples, of which here is a simple one. A young pupil, asked what will be the length of the longest side of a right-angled isosceles triangle, of which each of the shorter sides is one inch, will often answer "Two inches" with complete confidence. The teacher can at once create doubt, which he can then use in various ways according to the aim of the lesson, by drawing a square, divided into two triangles by a diagonal, on the blackboard, and asking : Which is the quicker way of getting from this corner of this square field to the opposite corner—

along these two sides, or along this path ? (indicating the diagonal).

As a lesson proceeds the teacher is continually both checking and furthering the understanding of his pupils by means of questions. Reference to this kind of questioning is made in later Sections. Questioning often reveals pupils' misconceptions, and is especially valuable as a means of detecting misunderstanding of the meanings of words. Teachers also, like all speakers, often use what might be called " rhetorical questions ", questions, that is to say, whose chief function is to secure continuity in a narrative, or to give the narrative more force, and which are either immediately answered by the teacher himself or are left unanswered.[1] " When the Spanish ships were collected in Calais harbour, what did the English do ? " This trivial question, part of a narrative of the Spanish Armada, illustrates the kind of question to which I refer. The pupils, we may suppose, have not previously heard anything about the Armada, and they are not expected to give any answer to the question. The teacher, in fact, gives the answer at once : " They sent fire-ships into the harbour ". " Rhetorical questions " can generally be avoided, and the teacher of young pupils will often be well advised to avoid them. For, young children are

---

[1] The rhetorical question is frequently used in literature : " Shall the thing formed say to him that formed it, Why hast thou made me thus ? Hath not the potter power over the clay, of the same lump to make one vessel unto honour, and another unto dishonour ? " (*Romans*, ix, 19-20.)

" O why should fate sic pleasure have
Life's dearest bonds untwining ?
Or why sae sweet a flower as love
Depend on fortune's shining ? "

(Burns, *Poortith Cauld*.)

Although these literary examples conform to the usual meaning of the term "rhetorical question", the question about the Armada does not. I have, in fact, given the term "rhetorical question" a some-what wider meaning than it usually carries.

inclined to regard every question spoken by the teacher as a request for an answer, and their replies to a series of rhetorical questions may break the continuity of the teacher's narrative. This would not be worth mentioning but for the fact that many inexperienced teachers make an undue use of rhetorical questions; they form what might be called the "interrogative habit", constantly asking questions to which they expect no answer, which in fact they do not wish the pupils to answer. Students training for teaching will sometimes in their practice lessons give a long narrative, almost every other sentence of which is interrogative in form.

We may now summarize the principal uses of questioning in teaching. The question may be used as a *test*, either to gauge the effects of previous teaching, or to provide the teacher with enough understanding of the extent of his pupils' knowledge to enable him to teach them effectively. Again, questions may be used to arouse interest. This is often effected by inducing the pupils, through a question, to look at some familiar thing from a new point of view ; or, what often comes to the same thing, by asking a question which makes the pupils critical of a belief they have hitherto confidently held. Further, in the course of exposition a teacher must constantly employ questions to check the understanding of his pupils, and by suitable questions asked at the right time he may assist their thinking and help them to see in what direction the lesson is tending. These various uses of questioning will now be considered in more detail.

2. *Oral Tests*

Before we turn to questioning as a teaching [1] device a few practical details of the process of oral testing must

---

[1] This use of the word " teaching " as an adjective, now commonly found in writings on education, is not happy ; but it enables the writer to avoid the ugly words " pedagogical " and " methodological ".

L

be considered.   Oral testing usually takes less time than testing by written examination, and it has other advantages. Thus it enables the teacher to deal with obscurities of understanding as they arise in the pupils' answers ; and it gives many pupils, especially young pupils, who find difficulty in expressing themselves in writing, more chance of free expression than they have in a written test.   But the oral test needs careful handling.   The teacher should, whenever possible, prepare his questions beforehand,[1] since the construction of a good series of questions is not a matter that can safely be left to his inspiration in the classroom.   In the distribution of the questions over the pupils he has some choice of procedure.   Each question should be put to the whole class.   If the questions require but brief answers the teacher can make sure that the whole class is attempting to answer them by requiring every pupil to write down the answers.   This is generally the best procedure in a test in mental arithmetic.   Such a test is not, however, properly speaking an oral test. Alternatively the teacher, having stated a question to the class as a whole, can allow one or two pupils to answer, passing over wrong answers without comment until he has received a few sufficiently correct answers.   In order to sample the attainments of the class by this second procedure the teacher must, of course, obtain answers, to one question or another, both from the more advanced and from the backward pupils.   Since we are here dealing with practical details,[2] it will be well to mention a further

[1] If (in, for example, a test in mental arithmetic) the teacher invents his questions as he goes along, and gives the whole series before he considers the answers (the pupils having written these down), he must be careful to make a note of each question as he gives it !   The back of the blackboard may be used for this purpose.

[2] The experienced teacher, if he finds the above remarks trite, is cordially invited to skip them.   This Section, and much of this chapter, is addressed to students in training and young teachers rather than to those of more experience.

precaution that should be taken in oral questioning. If only a few pupils volunteer to answer a question, it is often better to reword the question than to accept any answers from these few ; and it is nearly always better to do that than to allow any of the volunteers to give a lengthy wrong answer, in that way wasting the time and confusing the minds of the rest of the class.

3. *Use of Questioning to create Motive*

Whilst the innumerable questions of the young child are due to insatiable curiosity, the teacher often uses questions in order to *arouse* curiosity. A single question, if it presents a familiar thing in a new light, may suffice to arouse that active " interest " which is the emotional side of an effort to improve understanding. But there is an important condition that must usually be satisfied if a question is to stimulate reflection. If the teacher asks a series of disconnected questions, as is sometimes done in what are called " General Knowledge lessons ", requiring explanations of commonly occurring phenomena (*e.g.*, Why does a cut apple turn brown ? Why does a mirror become moist when breathed upon ? Why are flowers removed from a sick room at night ? etc.), answering each question himself as soon as he has asked it, he will arouse but a feeble interest. He is, in fact, *wasting* the questions, each of which should be introduced as a link in a *connected series of inquiries ;* each of which, moreover, if introduced at all, should be made a subject for *reflection on the part of the pupils*. Questions which are immediately answered by the teacher are merely " rhetorical ". The question about the flowers in the sick room, for example, if put to a class totally unacquainted with botany, is a question of this kind. Being quite beyond the reach of the pupils, it cannot stimulate reflection, and it will rarely arouse interest. We have reiterated the assertion that, from a psychological point of view, a question is a situation experienced as in some way incomplete. In order that a question may be actively appreciated as such, the questionee must have some idea, however ill-defined, of the kind of " completion " that is possible. Hence if the question about the moist mirror is introduced *at an appropriate point in a course of study of physics*, it may, although none of the pupils can answer it at the time, at once arouse a profitable curiosity which, if directed by further questions and other aids (such as references by the teacher to relevant facts with which the pupils are already acquainted), lead the pupils to explore the problem for themselves.

The use of questioning in the introduction of a new topic may be illustrated by the following account of the beginning of a first lesson on the Theorem of Pythagoras[1]:—

(The teacher has a piece of apparatus, which the reader should sketch from the following description before he reads further. Two wooden, or metal strips, AC and BC, are pivoted at C. AC is three inches long, BC is four inches. A string, attached to A, passes through a pinhole at B. Thus the angle ACB and the side AB can be varied at will.)

Teacher (starting with the strips open at any acute angle).—If I increase this angle (pointing to ACB) what will happen to AB ?

Pupil.—AB will increase.

T. (Shows that this answer is correct. Then closes the angle by pulling the free end of the string.)—What is happening to AB ?

P.—It is decreasing. (If this answer is not given, the

<hr>
[1] See p. 118.

teacher should point out that the string is running through the pinhole, so that AB is evidently getting shorter.)

T.—And the angle is——?

P.—Decreasing.

T.—The bigger the angle, the bigger the——?

P.—Side.

T.—What is the least value of the angle ?

P.—Nought degrees.

T.—And the greatest ?

P.—A hundred and eighty degrees.

T.—What is the least length AB can have ?

P.—One inch.

T.—And the greatest ?

P.—Seven inches.

T.—When the angle is 0°, AB is one inch, and when the angle is 180°, AB is seven inches. What do you think AB will be when the angle is 90° ?

The two commonest answers are three and a half and four inches. In either case the teacher draws the triangle on the blackboard and numbers the sides according to the answer given. It is at once seen that neither answer can be correct. The question is then put : How can we find what the length of AB is ? A discussion ensues in which the teacher shows that measurement is not a possible method of settling the matter exactly. In each of the extreme positions, when the angle was 0° and 180° respectively, it was possible to *calculate* the corresponding length of AB. Can calculation be applied to the right-angled triangle ? It is possible to develop from that point onwards a proof of Pythagoras's Theorem of such a character that the introductory discussion of the varying triangle is seen by the pupils to have been a very proper preliminary to the proof. But space prevents us from continuing here. There are other good methods of leading pupils up to this Theorem. The chief merits of the method given above are that it at once introduces the pupil to what is for him a new idea, namely the idea of applying *calculation* to the solution of problems that have hitherto been solved by drawing ; and that it is possible, in the proof to which the method leads, for the pupils to make each step in the reasoning with very little assistance from the teacher.

The *apparent irrelevance* of a question to the matter under discussion in class may sometimes excite curiosity, but such a question must quickly be followed by explanation or illuminated by further questions, lest the sustained unintelligibility of the procedure render it ineffective. After his class has examined a map of the Netherlands, observing particularly that much of the region is below sea-level, the teacher may put the apparently foolish question : Do rivers flow down, or up, to sea-level ?   He follows this up with the question : Then what can you say about the level of a river-bed before the river reaches the sea ?   If, when the obvious answer that the bed must be above sea-level is obtained, the teacher now asks the pupils to follow the course of the Rhine across the Netherlands, he will thereby put a further question (which he need not put into words) : How is it possible for the Rhine to reach the sea across land which is below sea-level ?   And so is reached the conclusion, of such importance in the geography of the Netherlands, that the river-banks must be at a higher level than the surrounding land.

4. *The Wording of Questions*

Since children often find difficulty in carrying in mind other than short and simple sentences, the teacher of young pupils should use words economically in questioning.

If a question cannot be stated in few words, it will usually be advisable to break it up into two or more shorter questions.   It is not unnecessary to advise beginners in teaching to speak their questions slowly, and generally to repeat them.   And there is another precaution that should be mentioned here.   It is the taking care that questions are free from ambiguity.   The teacher must not be content with knowing what answer he wants the pupils to give ;   the pupils must know what kind of answer he wants !   Thus the question :   What do the people of Ireland do ?   is not certain to produce the answer expected by the student who put that question when practising in a school ;   the answer, namely, that the people of Ireland grow potatoes !   Nor could another student expect his pupils to put on the following question the very special meaning he intended :   How do you know that $2 \times 6 = 12$?   His subsequent explanation showed that he had hoped the pupils would produce the argument that, since 6 is twice 3, and 12 is four times 3, therefore 12 must be twice 6.   With this vague question in arithmetic may be compared the following from geometry :—

There is a straight road to the station.   Or you can go by a straight road to the post-office, and then by another straight road to the station.   Which is the shorter way to the station ?   And why ?

The answer expected is one that only a sophisticated child would give :   that, namely, the direct route is shorter " because two sides of a triangle are together greater than the third ".   Here we have a flagrant example of the kind of illegitimate question that may sometimes be asked with the intention of illuminating an element of common sense. It is as true to say that the straight road is shorter, because it is straight, as it is to say that the indirect route is longer because " two sides of a triangle are together greater than the third ". That proposition is, in fact, nothing more than an abstract statement of the intuitive conception of straightness which is held by men and animals alike. The child who justifies the short cut on the plea that one side of a triangle is less than the sum of the other two is not showing any more understanding of the matter than the dog who runs straight across a field rather than along two sides of it.

5. *Wordless Questions*

Interrogative situations may often be created in the course of teaching without the asking of verbally stated questions. It is often possible, for example, to ask questions by merely pointing to parts of a map, diagram or model. Such dumb show is often more effective than the corresponding series of oral questions would be. But the value of such procedures can only be appreciated when they are observed in skilful teaching, and no attempt will be made to describe them here. The reader can doubtless think of numerous questions that may be asked with the sole aid of a wall-map and pointer, or by means of a geometrical diagram. By the manipulation of apparatus in front of a class questions may be both put and answered with little or no speech from the teacher. When, for example, with the apparatus described above for the introduction of the Theorem of Pythagoras, the teacher has asked for the length of AB (one inch) in the "closed" position of the strips, if he opens the angle ACB to 180°, and then pauses, his action will be taken by most pupils as tantamount to the question : What is the length of AB *now ?* Indeed a well-timed pause in the teacher's speech often quite clearly puts a question to the class, and at other times a mere gesture may serve the same purpose.

6. *A Plea for the Oral Lesson*

The widespread advocacy of " individual work ", which is a very welcome feature of present-day educational programmes, creates some danger that the importance of the oral lesson may be underestimated. Whilst the pupil can conduct much of his education in the company of books he needs also the inspiration that only a teacher can give : and he needs to be taught as a member of a *group*. Education by inquiry, in library or laboratory, is not more important than the education by discussion which is possible in class teaching. If teachers have hitherto given their pupils, in oral lessons, much that the pupils should have been allowed to take for themselves from books, they can yet give much that is not to be found in books. The chief gifts of the oral lesson should be inspiration and the opportunity of free discussion. It is only half true that " the true university is a collection of books ". But so to describe " the true school " would be still less true.

In making this, perhaps unnecessary, plea for the oral lesson, I should be misunderstood if it were supposed that I failed to recognize how much more use could be made advantageously of methods of " individual work " than is commonly made at the present time. But it is important to consider carefully the conditions for the success of such methods. The chief conditions are : a supply of suitable books ; and desire for inquiry, and some skill in unaided inquiry, on the part of the pupils. Upon what does skill in inquiry mainly depend ? The art of study consists essentially in propounding questions to oneself and then trying to solve them. . This rhythm of question and answer runs throughout all learning and all teaching. We may start the study of a new subject without any clear consciousness of the problems and experiences it involves, but with a feeling of adventure. The explorer of a strange country, however, soon finds his quest gaining definiteness —he is on the banks of a river and must follow them to the source ; he sees a peak in the distance and cannot rest until he has reached it ; he finds the remains of a human settlement, and is set wondering what kind of people lit the fire that left those ashes. So, the student who knows his craft, has not read the first page of his book before his general motive of wanting to know something about the subject is replaced by, or accompanied by, aims of solving specific problems. Learning how to study consists largely in learning how to create problems. That is to say, the student's first need is skill in the art of interrogation. We have seen in this chapter of how great use a teacher may be in presenting to pupils problems that they would not discover for themselves. Whether it be by word of mouth in class, or by printed word in a textbook, one of the teacher's principal functions must always be to ask the right question at the right time.

The process of thinking may be viewed from many standpoints and described in many ways. From one point of view such activity, whether we are considering an individual's solution of a single problem or the growth of his mind throughout his life, appears to be a process of development from experiences that are incomplete to experiences that are in some way more complete. We may say that " the appreciation of a question," in the broadest sense of the phrase, is the initial phase of any process of cognitive development. This initial experience may be capable of much or of little growth ; it may be capable of growth along only one or two lines, all leading inevitably to the same end, as when we solve a mathematical problem ; or it may be capable of development in many ways, as when we start thinking with no more clearly defined question than, for example, What is the nature of mind ?

We may bring this sketch of some of the principles of interrogation to a close by expressing the hope that it will have created in the reader's mind an " initial experience " capable of development along lines that will lead towards the solution of many problems of cardinal importance in education.

INDEX

Words used in a special sense are in italics.
References to definitions are in italics.

ABILITIES, 70-2
Ability, 113 ; average, 34-5 ; effective, 41-2 ; general, 36, 133 ; mathematical, 133 ; and knowledge, 131-5
Abstraction, 12, 46, 51, 74-5
Addition, 41-2, 69
Algebra, 44-5
Analysis, 12, 33
Argument, of test, *41* fn., 72-5
Arithmetic, 44, 78, 99, 162, 167
Association, 32
Attention, 77
Attitude, 126-31

BADMINTON, 19
Ballard, P. B., 95 fn., 102 fn., 105
Behaviour, 5-7, 24, 25, 57
Belief, 113
Bias, 93, 145
Binet-Simon Tests, *see* Tests
Blind writing, 121
Burt, C., 105
Butler, Samuel, 132 fn.

CAPACITY, 78, 132
Categories, psychological, 12, 49-50
Chance, 29
Chemistry, 100, 135
Chess, 10
Confusion, 125
Correlation, 49, 68-72
Cramming, 128

DEGREES, of correctness, 29, 63
Description, modes of, 5-8
Difficulty, 29, 30, 53
Dispositions, 5
Distance, *61*
Doubt, creation of, 159

EBBINGHAUS, *see* Test
Education, 127, 128, 169
Eduction, 36-7, 52, 68
Enduring qualities, 2-5

Error, assessment of, 123 ; *of definition*, *75*, 76-8, 84 ; in physics, 75, 77 ; in testing, 75-9
Essays, 63, 91-2, 107-8, 112
Examinations, Chs. IV, V *passim* ; aims of, 88-90 ; criticism of, 93-5; as incentives, 130 ; *indication* of, 89 ; " new," 95, 101-7, 140, 146 ; in philosophy and psychology, 119-20 ; syllabuses of, 130-1
Examiners, competence of, 97-8 ; discrepancy between, 96-100
Examining process, stages of, 90-3
Expression, 24-32, 57, 123-6

FACT, and *precision*, 141
Factors, common, 66-7, 70-2 ; determining, 46 ; interference, 76-8 ; theory of two, 71
Fatigue, 78
Fear, 16
French Revolution, 141-2

GEOGRAPHY, 100, 123, 166
Geometry, 164-6, 167-8
Gordon, Hugh, 41 fn.
Guessing, 104, 155-6
Guidance, in questions, 152-3

HISTORY, 91, 115, 135, 138
Huntingdon and Cushing, 148, 149

IMAGERY, visual, 48-9
Indication, *16-21*, 32-40, 44-9, 76, 118-9 ; *primary*, 37
Indicative power, *see* Questions
Individual differences, 8-12, 53
Individual work, 169-70
Information, 114, 122
Insight, 28, 50, 117-8
Instructions, 32, 38-40, 78-9
Intelligence, 18, 20, 73-4, 80 ; tests of, *see* Tests
Interest, 129, 161, 163
Introspection, 24, 49, 50, 100
Invention, 51